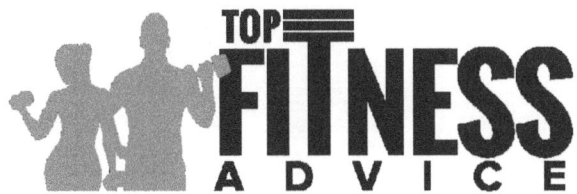

HEALTHY HABITS VOL. 3

119 Everyday Habits You WISH You KNEW to Lose Weight, Live Healthy, Feel Energized, Live Longer & Sleep Well!

LINDA WESTWOOD

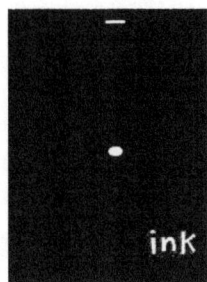

First published in 2015 by Venture Ink Publishing

Copyright © Top Fitness Advice 2019

All rights reserved.

No part of this book may be reproduced in any form without permission in writing from the author. No part of this publication may be reproduced or transmitted in any form or by any means, mechanic, electronic, photocopying, recording, by any storage or retrieval system, or transmitted by email without the permission in writing from the author and publisher.

Requests to the publisher for permission should be addressed to publishing@ventureink.co

For more information about the contents of this book or questions to the author, please contact Linda Westwood at linda@topfitnessadvice.com

Disclaimer

This book provides wellness management information in an informative and educational manner only, with information that is general in nature and that is not specific to you, the reader. The contents of this book are intended to assist you and other readers in your personal wellness efforts. Consult your physician regarding the applicability of any information provided in this book to you.

Nothing in this book should be construed as personal advice or diagnosis, and must not be used in this manner. The information provided about conditions is general in nature. This information does not cover all possible uses, actions, precautions, side-effects, or interactions of medicines, or medical procedures. The information in this book should not be considered as complete and does not cover all diseases, ailments, physical conditions, or their treatment.

You should consult with your physician before beginning any exercise, weight loss, or health care program. This book should not be used in place of a call or visit to a competent health-care professional. You should consult a health care professional before adopting any of the suggestions in this book or before drawing inferences from it.

Any decision regarding treatment and medication for your condition should be made with the advice and consultation of a qualified health care professional. If you have, or suspect you have, a health-care problem, then you should immediately contact a qualified health care professional for treatment.

No Warranties: The author and publisher don't guarantee or warrant the quality, accuracy, completeness, timeliness, appropriateness or suitability of the information in this book, or of any product or services referenced in this book.

The information in this book is provided on an "as is" basis and the author and publisher make no representations or warranties of any kind with respect to this information. This book may contain inaccuracies, typographical errors, or other errors.

Liability Disclaimer: The publisher, author, and other parties involved in the creation, production, provision of information, or delivery of this book specifically disclaim any responsibility, and shall not be held liable for any damages, claims, injuries, losses, liabilities, costs, or obligations including any direct, indirect, special, incidental, or consequences damages (collectively known as "Damages") whatsoever and howsoever caused, arising out of, or in connection with the use or misuse of the site and the information contained within it, whether such Damages arise in contract, tort, negligence, equity, statute law, or by way of other legal theory.

Table of Contents

Disclaimer	3
Who is this book for?	13
What will this book teach you?	13
Introduction	14
Everyday Habit #1: Slow It Down!	16
Everyday Habit #2: Stop Eating After Dinner	21
Everyday Habit #3: If You Eat, Don't Cheat	23
Everyday Habit #4: Cut This Out & Lose Weight FASTER Than Before!	28
Everyday Habit #5: Make Sleep a Priority	30
Everyday Habit #6: Cut the Caffeine	36
Everyday Habit #7: Avoid Alcohol & Tobacco	40
Everyday Habit #8: This Will STOP Evening Food Cravings	43
Everyday Habit #9: Don't Confuse Thirst for Hunger	44
Everyday Habit #10: The CURE to Night Binges Fits in Your Pocket!	47
Everyday Habit #11: Take an After-Dinner Walk	48
Everyday Habit #12: Turn off the T.V.	52
Everyday Habit #13: Curb Cravings with Nutrition (Part I)	55

Everyday Habit #14: Curb Cravings with Nutrition (Part II)	58
Everyday Habit #15: Establish Food-Free Zones	60
Everyday Habit #16: Know What Your Body Is Actually Telling You	63
Everyday Habit #17: Make After-Dinner Snacking Hard Work	68
Everyday Habit #18: "Serving Size" Is Not Just a Suggestion	69
Everyday Habit #19: Start Snack-Free Shopping	70
Everyday Habit #20: Track Your Progress and Stay Motivated	74
Everyday Habit #21: Take the 30-Day Weight Loss Challenge	76
Bonus Tips	78
Everyday Habit #22: Focus on Vegetables	85
Everyday Habit #23: Increase This & See Results Immediately!	87
Everyday Habit #24: Add Healthy Oil to Every Meal	88
Everyday Habit #25: Balance Your Protein and Carbs	90
Everyday Habit #26: Take a Fish Oil Supplement	92
Everyday Habit #27: The FUN Habit with MANY Benefits	94
Everyday Habit #28: Eat Dessert	96
Everyday Habit #29: The Easiest Alternative to Working Out	98
Everyday Habit #30: Binge Drink on Water!	101
Everyday Habit #31: Reduce Refined Sugars in Your Diet	103

Everyday Habit #32: The Wonders of a Single Cup of Green Tea Daily   105

Everyday Habit #33: Don't Ditch Breakfast   107

Everyday Habit #34: Sleep Enough!   108

Everyday Habit #35: Eat Colorful Meals   110

Everyday Habit #36: Eat Negative Calorie Snack Foods   111

Everyday Habit #37: Consume Healthy Fats Regularly   112

Everyday Habit #38: Create Your Own Flavored Water   114

Everyday Habit #39: Strength Training Boosts Fat Loss!   115

Everyday Habit #40: This Habit Will Make You Eat LESS   116

Everyday Habit #41: Break Your Weight Loss Goals into Manageable Pieces   118

Everyday Habit #42: Pack Your Lunch   118

Everyday Habit #43: Use Smaller Plates   119

Everyday Habit #44: Reduce or Remove Red Meat from Your Diet   120

Everyday Habit #45: Eat Slower   121

Everyday Habit #46: Snack on Vegetables and Nuts   122

Everyday Habit #47: Meditate Daily   123

Everyday Habit #48: Avoid Artificial Sweeteners   124

Everyday Habit #49: Replace One Meal a Day with a Protein Shake   125

Everyday Habit #50: Take a Multi-Vitamin Daily	127
Everyday Habit #51: Don't Forget Fish	128
Everyday Habit #52: Avoid Places You Used to Eat At	129
Everyday Habit #53: Avoid Empty Liquid Calories	131
Everyday Habit #54: Try Yoga	132
Everyday Habit #55: Eat Vegetarian Once a Week	134
Everyday Habit #56: Limit Your Sodium Intake	136
Everyday Habit #57: Cook Meals at Home When Possible	137
Everyday Habit #58: Eat All of Your Meals as a Family	139
Everyday Habit #59: Incorporate Chia Seeds into Your Diet	140
Everyday Habit #60: Negative Calorie Foods Cheat Sheet	142
Everyday Habit #61: Know Your Carbohydrates	146
Bonus Tips	149
Extra Bonus Advice!	155
Everyday Habit #62: Punch Something!	156
Everyday Habit #63: This Habit Will Surprise You!	160
Everyday Habit #64: Walk Around Barefoot (At Home)	165
Everyday Habit #65: Take More Naps!	166
Everyday Habit #66: Use A Neti Pot	169
Everyday Habit #67: Clean Cash	171

Everyday Habit #68: Shut the Lid! 172

Everyday Habit #69: Natural Migraine Destroyer 175

Everyday Habit #70: Drink Chocolate Milk! 177

Everyday Habit #71: Something You May Not Want to Hear ... 179

Everyday Habit #72: Surprising Benefit of Dental Hygiene ... 183

Everyday Habit #73: Adults Only 185

Everyday Habit #74: Weigh Yourself Regularly 187

Everyday Habit #75: Plan Your Meals 188

Everyday Habit #76: Plan & Carry Healthy Snacks 189

Everyday Habit #77: Find Lower Calorie Alternatives 190

Everyday Habit #78: Eat Slowly 191

Everyday Habit #79: Stop Drinking Calories 193

Everyday Habit #80: Have Patience 194

Everyday Habit #81: Aim to Exercise for Just 10 Minutes A Day ... 195

Everyday Habit #82: Eat Real Food 196

Everyday Habit #83: Use Smaller Dishes 198

Everyday Habit #84: Order Your Coffee Black 199

Everyday Habit #85: Make Walking After Dinner A Habit ... 200

Everyday Habit #86: Eat Salad Dressing On The Side 202

Everyday Habit #87: Stop Ordering Appetizers & Desserts ... 203

Everyday Habit #88: Eat Before You Get Really Hungry	204
Everyday Habit #89: Always Pack Your Lunch	206
Everyday Habit #90: Deal with Stress	208
Everyday Habit #91: Sit Down to Eat	209
Everyday Habit #92: Cut Down Your TV Time	210
Everyday Habit #93: Eat on A Schedule	210
Everyday Habit #94: Keep A Food Diary	211
Everyday Habit #95: Opt for The Stairs	212
Everyday Habit #96: Park Further from The Door	212
Everyday Habit #97: Never Skip Meals	213
Everyday Habit #98: Slow Down with The Carbs	213
Everyday Habit #99: Less Meat, More Grains & Vegetables	214
Everyday Habit #100: Start Eating Soup Regularly	215
Everyday Habit #101: Don't Bring Junk Food Home	216
Everyday Habit #102: Always Shop with A Full Belly	216
More Bonus Tips!	217
Everyday Habit #103: Don't Retire	218
Everyday Habit #104: Get At Least 6 Hours of Sleep	219
Everyday Habit #105: MOVE!	225
Everyday Habit #106: Start Jogging	231

Everyday Habit #107: NEVER Forget This — 235

Everyday Habit #108: Cut Out The CRAP! — 241

Everyday Habit #109: Reduce Sun Time — 246

Everyday Habit #110: The MOST Important Drink — 248

Everyday Habit #111: Floss Daily — 250

Everyday Habit #112: Breakfast Really is the MOST Important Meal — 253

Everyday Habit #113: The RIGHT Breakfast — 254

Everyday Habit #114: Eat Food, Not Supplements — 258

Everyday Habit #115: Go with The Flow — 260

Everyday Habit #116: Build Habits — 264

Everyday Habit #117: Socialize — 265

Everyday Habit #118: Cut Your TV Time — 267

Everyday Habit #119: Eat Some Nuts Every Day — 271

Everyday Habit #120: Consume LESS Red Meat — 273

Everyday Habit #121: Eat More Sushi — 276

Everyday Habit #122: Eat Chocolate! — 278

Everyday Habit #123: Try to Be Happier — 279

Everyday Habit #124: Get on Your Feet — 282

Everyday Habit #125: Don't Overeat — 283

Everyday Habit #126: Have "Fun" Time – Regularly!	284
Conclusion	286
Final Words	288

Would you prefer to listen to my book, rather than read it?

Download the audiobook version for free!

If you go to the special link below and sign up to Audible as a new customer, you can get the audiobook version of my book completely free.

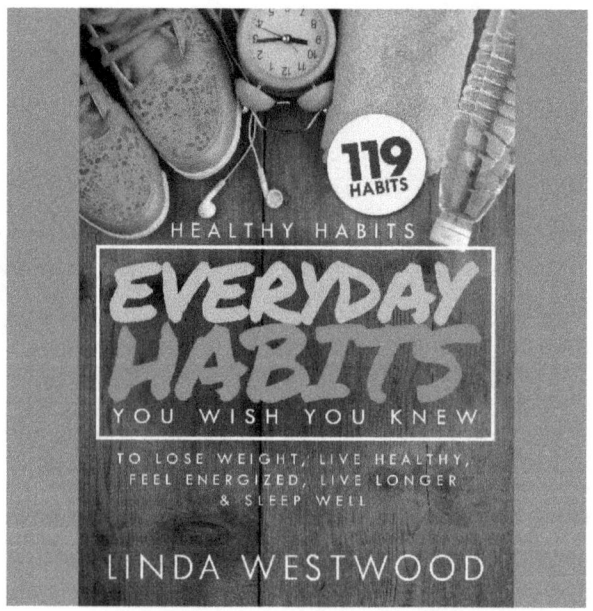

Go here to get your audiobook version for free:

TopFitnessAdvice.com/go/everyday

Who is this book for?

Do you feel that your binges and cravings ruin your diet? Are you struggling to stick to healthy habits and lose weight? Do you want to feel healthy and energized all day long? Are you one of those people who *know* what to do, but struggle to *actually do* it?

Then this book is for you!

I am going to share with you some of the MOST effective everyday habits that you can add into your life to lose weight, feel great and sleep well! I have given you a simple action plan at the end of each chapter so you can implement each habit very easily!

Also, you don't have to be overweight to benefit from these habits. Yes, they help you lose weight, but they also help you live a healthy life, live longer, as well as sleep well at night!

What will this book teach you?

This book is not like others! It doesn't just contain generic advice that we all already know, but actual everyday habits that have been identified to INCREASE weight loss, IMPROVE sleep quality, BOOST longevity, and LEAD to a more healthy life!

Some of these habits are very simple and you can begin implementing them from tonight, and some are a little more difficult, in that you will need to practice them more!

I will also share with you why each of these habits work and are so effective – along with a simple action plan to help get you started and on your way to lasting success!

Introduction

To begin, let's take a look at healthy habits you can add into your evening routine, and how you can live longer, live healthy, and sleep well at night. A lot of people will tell you that getting a good fresh start to the day is the most important part of leading a happy, healthy life. But the secret to getting that fresh start is building the right habits the evening or day before.

The day before (especially the evening) is your time to decompress and rejuvenate yourself. It is your time to strengthen your resolve and recharge your batteries so that tomorrow morning, you actually wake up feeling fresh and ready to take on the day. Your daily routine can make or break your weight loss plan. Even after spending the whole day staying strong and sticking to a healthy diet, it could all be undone by your midnight snacking in front of the television when you get home at night.

Snacking—especially when you're snacking on junk food right before you go to sleep—can pack on more calories than you even realize. And once you fall asleep, your metabolism drops into low gear and ends up just storing most of those extra calories as fat. So if you've been trying to lose weight but have found yourself stagnating and unable to burn those finicky pounds, it might be because your evening habits are holding you back (and holding the weight on).

Unfortunately, most diet plans and health advice focus on what you should be doing in the mornings and during the day. But after dinnertime, they've got little to no advice. At most, they'll simply say, "don't snack after dinner" or "get a good night's sleep" as if just telling yourself to do it will actually make it happen.

Almost every healthy weight loss habit is easier said than done but that doesn't mean they are impossible. This book is here to give you real advice that you can really use. It won't just tell you "don't snack after dinner"; it will give you a solid action plan for *how* to undo that nasty post-dinner snacking habit. You'll get in depth details and step-by-step advice for eliminating the bad habits that are holding you back and cultivating the good habits that will help you finally shed that extra weight once and for all.

A healthy and rejuvenating end to the day is just as important as that fresh start. Speed up your weight loss by cutting out those weight gain causing habits and replace them with effective yet simple weight loss strategies. We won't pretend it's easy but it *is* easier than you think especially if you know exactly what you can do to accomplish it. There are many habits in this book. Each of them will help you lose weight faster. But if you really want to increase your chances of losing weight and keeping it off, don't overwhelm yourself by deciding to start doing all the habits at once.

Take them a step at a time. Give each habit the time it deserves to become fully incorporated into your daily routine. If you give each habit time, it will actually become a full habit, meaning you won't have to constantly remind yourself to do it and you won't find yourself struggling to keep up with it. You'll actually change the way you do things and finally get rid of those unhealthy habits that have been packing on pounds faster than you can burn them off.

So, read through each step, learn why it works, and then read the action plan for how to actually incorporate it into your routine. In addition to individual tips for adopting each habit, you'll get a sample calendar for a 30-day challenge in the last chapter. This calendar will help you adopt all 21 habits in a way that will help make sure you stick with them for the long term. Each habit from this book will help you either cut more calories or burn more calories so the more habits you pack on, the more pounds you are going to see drop off!

Everyday Habit #1

Slow It Down!

One of the most important habits you can practice is eating slowly. You need to take your time with food rather than just shoveling it down while you drive to work. Eating slowly might not seem like it would change how many calories you eat, just how long it takes you to eat them. But it does actually help you reduce the number of calories and keep you feeling full between meals. Multiple studies have been done which show that people who eat slowly also eat less.

In one study, the participants who ate slowly ate an average of 100 calories less than the participants who ate quickly. In another study, participants were all given the same amount of ice cream. Some were told to eat it in 5 minutes and others were told to eat it in 30 minutes. Those who spent 30 minutes eating the ice cream had a higher concentration of hormones in their stomach that caused them to feel fuller for longer. This means that the physical signal (the hormones) to feel full will be stronger if you eat slowly so you feel full sooner and you keep feeling full longer.

So, if you make slow eating a habit, you'll eat fewer calories in one meal and avoid adding more calories between meals. This habit alone can dramatically reduce the total number of calories you eat in a day, which will help you lose weight much more quickly. Fast eating not only causes you to eat more total calories, it doesn't let your body produce enough of the hormone that makes you feel full. Without that hormone, you could eat 1,000 calories and still feel hungry enough to eat a horse because the full feeling you should have just isn't there.

On the other hand, if you eat slowly, you could eat a 300-calorie meal and be so full that you feel as if you *did* just eat a horse. Plus, that full feeling will last for hours after you've eaten so you're less likely to want to snack between meals. The bottom line: eating *less* food can make you feel *more* satisfied if you eat it slowly. But there are even more benefits to eating slowly than just eating less and feeling fuller. You also get more pleasure from your food.

When you eat slowly, you are giving yourself the time to savor and enjoy every single bite. You get the full experience of the food on your plate and the full range of flavors it has to offer. Getting more pleasure out of your mealtime is more important than you might think. Our brains have evolved to seek out pleasure and avoid pain.

In the case of food, our brains are seeking out the pleasure of eating and avoiding the pain of feeling hunger. So, when you don't take the time to enjoy your meal, your brain isn't getting the pleasure signal it's looking for which means it's going to keep looking for more food even though you've literally just eaten.

At the physiological level, feeling pleasure releases certain neurotransmitters and hormones in the body. These neurotransmitters and hormones are what give you the physical sensations that come with pleasure: relaxed muscles, reduced pain, lower blood pressure, and the emotional and physical feeling of wellbeing. This same pleasure process that is making you feel more relaxed is responsible for turning your metabolism. That means that simply taking the time to enjoy your meal can increase your metabolism.

If that's not enough to convince you, the hormones that make you feel stressed actually slow down your metabolism. So, eating quickly and feeling rushed while you eat can actually slow down your metabolism. At the physical level, stress hormones are your body's way of knowing that it needs to start planning for a worst-case scenario. It slows down digestion and stores more of the calories as fat because it thinks it should prepare for a famine. Your body can't tell the difference between stress about work and stress about not having enough food. So, when you feel stressed or guilty while eating, you are causing your body to store fat. When you feel pleasure while eating, you are telling your body that everything is fine and there is no need to store any fat for later.

So, to sum it all up, eating slowly and enjoying your meal has three powerful weight loss effects in your body:

1. Decreased total calorie intake
2. Increased production of the hormone that makes you feel full
3. Increased metabolism

So, you eat less, you feel full for longer, and you burn the calories more quickly. All of that happens just because you took your time to eat and enjoy food!

Action Plan

Now that you know why it's so important to eat slowly and enjoy your meal, it's time to learn how you can actually start doing it. When you first start, it's going to be difficult to slow down your pace for the entire meal. You'll feel a little impatient and have a hard time resisting the impulse to just keep shoveling in bite after bite. But you can and should do it.

Since you want to increase pleasure as well, it might not be good to time yourself for each bite. It could just end up stressing you out. Instead, slow down by taking time to enjoy the food. Take one bite at a time. Put your fork or spoon down after you take the bite. Chew your food slowly and let it roll over your tongue. Be aware and consciously think about the different flavors and textures that you are experiencing. You can make a game out of it by trying to recognize every ingredient in the dish.

Is that a hint of rosemary you taste? Maybe there's a dash of cinnamon. Even if you made it yourself and already know every ingredient that is in it, try to actually recognize each ingredient that you added. Once you have swallowed the bite, take a sip of water—or wine, whatever you are drinking with your meal. Then, pick your fork back up and take the next bite. Take the time to experience and enjoy that one, too.

If you still find that you're having a hard time slowing down, there are actually apps available for your smartphone that help you eat slowly. Many of them are free so try downloading one and using it to help you get into the habit of slow eating. You might be thinking that eating slowly and enjoying your meal sounds great in theory but you just don't have the time to do it. If that's the case, make time. It's time to end the "working lunches", and wake up a little earlier to give yourself the time for a relaxing, enjoyable breakfast. You have read all the benefits of eating slowly and eating with pleasure so you know that it's worth making room in your schedule to do it.

Discover Scientifically-Proven "Shortcuts" & "Hacks" to Lose Weight FASTER (With Very Little Effort)

For this month only, you can get Linda's best-selling & most popular book absolutely free – *Weight Loss Secrets You NEED to Know*.

Get Your FREE Copy Here:
TopFitnessAdvice.com/Bonus

Discover scientifically-proven tips to help you lose weight faster and easier than ever before. With this book, readers were able to improve their weight loss results and fitness levels. So, it's highly recommended that you get this book, especially while it's free!

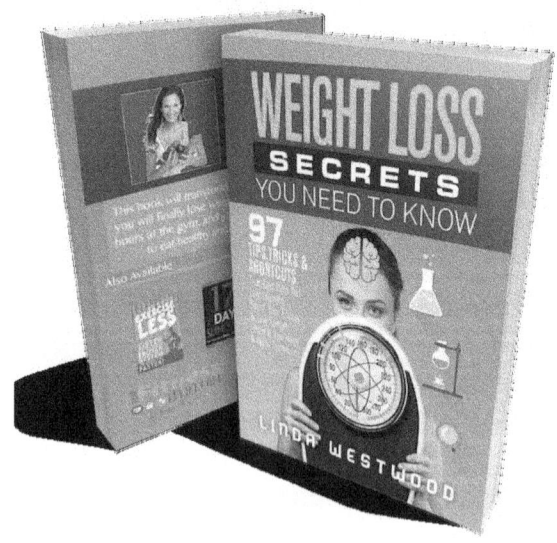

Get Your FREE Copy Here:
TopFitnessAdvice.com/Bonus

Everyday Habit #2

Stop Eating After Dinner

After-dinner snacking is the mortal enemy of any diet plan. It can undo all your efforts during the day to stick to your diet. It's not just the added calories but also the way you eat them and when you are eating them. In almost every case, snacking after dinner happens while you are sitting in front of the TV and not actually paying any attention to the food you are eating.

You have just finished reading through the first evening habit of eating slowly so you already know why it's so important to pay attention to your food while you eat it. You end up eating way more than you should and you hardly gain a fraction of the satisfaction you should be getting from it which means that your body doesn't have a chance to make the food-pleasure connection that you need in order to put cravings to rest.

Beyond that, it's also a lot of extra calories that you are taking on even though your dinner should have provided you with enough to get you through the rest of the night. You eat all these extra calories and then, what? You go to sleep—an activity that requires the bare minimum of calories. So you just took in a bunch of extra calories and then went on to do a low calorie activity. Your body has no other choice but to store those extra calories as fat.

In one study, participants were told to stop after dinner snacking for two weeks. They didn't change anything else at all about their eating habits or exercise habits. After two weeks, they lost 1 pound (just from cutting out evening snacks). But what is even more interesting about this study is the fact that after the two weeks, they were told to spend one week going back to their old routine of nighttime snacking.

In that one-week, they *gained* an average of 1.3 pounds. The only change was the evening snacking and they gained back all the weight they lost plus a little extra. This simple habit of cutting out after dinner snacks could cut about 250 calories from your daily total (depending on how many calories you tend to eat after dinner). That translates to about ½ a pound per week lost, just because you said no to your usual snack.

If you combine this with first habit, you could be cutting out more than 500 calories from your daily total every single day. Even if you make absolutely no other changes aside from these two things, that's already going to help you lose about 1 pound per week!

Action Plan

If you snack after dinner every night or almost every night, it's probably become a deeply engrained habit that will be hard to break but it's definitely worth the effort. So, what's the most simple and effective strategy for cutting out after dinner snacks? Just stop snacking after dinner! If you've got any willpower, just fight the urge. But if that strategy isn't working for you, get more creative with it: put up "closed" signs on the fridge or pantry after dinner to remind you that snack foods are off limits.

It sounds silly but having a big sign on the fridge when you go to open it makes it impossible to forget that you are not supposed to be getting any snacks. If the urge to snack is starting to feel like more than you can bear, do something else. Go for a walk (evening habit #11) or work on a craft. The need to feed will go down if you are keeping your mind and body actively involved in something else. You'll learn more about this when you learn about evening habits #11 and #12.

One of the best ways to keep from snacking is to not have snacks! Just don't buy them. Even if your kids throw a fit, they'll get over it eventually. Any food that can be eaten without any preparation (except for fruits and vegetables) should just be kept out of your kitchen. This might sound like a difficult adjustment to make but you'll learn more about later in this book. Evening habit #19 is all about snack-free shopping.

In fact, if post-meal snacks are a serious problem for you, many of the habits in this book will help you finally break the snacking routine and cut hundreds of calories from your daily total! So, keep on reading to learn more about how you can avoid snacking, cut total calories, and boost your metabolism so that you can finally lose the weight that's been burdening

Everyday Habit #3

If You Eat, Don't Cheat

No matter how strong your will power is, there are going to be some days when you simply can't avoid having a snack to help you make it through to the next meal. Sometimes, you just won't have the time to cook a full, balanced, healthy meal. Life can be hectic and you can't always devote as much time to your health as you would like to.

Luckily, there are some ways around this and there are habits you can build to make sure that even when you don't have time, you can still eat healthy and make sure you don't undo all the progress you have made. From planning your meals to snacking properly, you'll be able to keep your calorie count in a reasonable range and continue to lose weight no matter how busy you are.

The trick is to choose healthy, low calorie snacks that are satisfying to munch on without loading you up with extra calories. Your first line of defense, however, is making sure you have well-planned meals that are high in fiber and protein so that you can be sure you feel full between meals.

In the next section of this chapter (the action plan), you'll learn how to make a meal plan for the week that will fight cravings and keep your total number of calories low enough that you can shed the extra weight.cIf you still have cravings between meals even though you've planned them so well, there are some healthy snacks that you can keep in the house that won't break the calorie bank.

These are all foods that, after digestion, have a very minimal caloric impact. Some of these foods also have metabolism-boosting and appetite-controlling effects so they can help control your cravings and increase the rate at which you burn calories.

Of course, it's better not to snack at all because then your body will focus on burning the calories already stored as fat. But, if you absolutely have to munch on something, choose a minimal calorie food so that you aren't adding too many new calories.

Here are a few low-calorie foods you can snack on:

- Carrots
- Broccoli
- Spinach
- Radishes
- Cucumbers
- Melons (cantaloupe, honeydew, etc.)
- Peaches
- Pineapple
- Strawberries
- Mangoes
- Tangerines
- Garlic
- Onion
- Cinnamon
- Flax seed
- Cayenne pepper

- Chili powder

You'll get a few other healthy snack ideas in chapter 19 when you learn about snack-free shopping. At the end of the list, you got a few seasonings and some foods that you probably don't want to eat plain (like garlic or onion). Combine these foods together to create tasty, low-calorie meals.

For example, slice up a mango and dust it with cayenne and chili powder. It might sound strange but the spice of the cayenne and chili powder really complements the sweetness of the mango for an exciting flavor contrast. Toss some spinach with flax seeds, strawberries, and tangerines for a salad that is flavorful enough to be delicious without any diet-busting salad dressing. There are a lot of healthy options for snacking that won't add calories so there's no excuse for cheating on your diet just because your stomach is grumbling between meals.

Action Plan

As mentioned earlier, the best defense against between meal cravings is a well-designed meal plan and thorough preparation. If your weeks tend to be really busy and you often come home feeling too tired to prepare and cook a balanced, diet-friendly meal, then you should start preparing in advance. To do this, you'll need to make a menu for the entire week. This includes 3 meals for each day on every day of the week. Then, you'll write out your list of ingredients (including the exact amounts needed of each one) and go shopping.

Once you've got all your ingredients, you'll prepare all your meals for the week. Then all you have to do is store them in the meal-sized portions in the freezer. Throughout the week, you can come home, pull a meal out of the freezer and just reheat it for a completely balanced and satisfying meal without all the work.

Now, when you come home exhausted and hungry, you won't have to do any heavy cooking. You get to combine the convenience of processed, store-bought meals with the health and weight loss power of a fresh, home-cooked meal! It's best to do this on the weekend when you have more time. On Saturday or Sunday, spend the morning and afternoon planning, shopping, and cooking. Then, prepare to sit back and relax for the rest of the week!

As you plan your menu, make sure that you cover all your bases and come up with satisfying, healthy meals.

Here are some key things to consider as you plan:

1. The average person needs 25 to 30 grams of fiber daily. This means each meal should have about 10 grams of fiber.

    a. Whole grains, beans, legumes, and oatmeal are a few good options to meet your fiber requirements.

2. The average person needs about 50 grams of protein per day. So each meal should have roughly 16 or 17 grams of protein in it.

    a. Beans, legumes, egg yolks, nuts, yogurt, seeds, fish, seafood, and poultry are all healthy sources of protein that won't hurt your blood pressure or cholesterol levels (in fact, they will help lower both of these things).

3. The average person needs to eat about 30 grams of fat every day. This means about 10 grams per meal.

    a. As strange as it sounds, you do also need fat in your diet if you want to burn fat. Healthy fat (unsaturated fats) help fight high cholesterol and stabilize your blood glucose levels so that you don't get between meal cravings.

b. The key is to look for *unsaturated* fat. As you increase the amount of unsaturated fat, decrease the amount of saturated fats and Trans fats. Try to cut Trans fats out completely. Keep saturated fats down to around 3 to 5 grams.

c. Nuts, seeds, oils (olive, sesame, or coconut), fish, avocados, and olives are all great sources of unsaturated fats.

Each meal should contain something from each category. Make sure there are also at least one or two servings of fruits or vegetables in each meal. Fruits are especially good to include in your breakfast because the fructose (sugar) will provide an immediate energy boost while the protein, fiber, and fat from the rest of your breakfast will provide sustained and stable energy throughout the day. Your lunch should also have a couple servings of fruit as well to give you a quick boost while you wait for the protein, fiber, and fat to provide sustained energy. Avoid fruits or other simple sugars at dinner though, because you don't want a sharp spike in your blood glucose levels keeping you awake when it's time to go to bed. If you make sure that you have a wide variety of healthy whole foods throughout the day, you won't have to worry about counting calories or tediously tallying up all your vitamins and minerals.

The variety of different fruits, vegetables, grains, and proteins will help make sure that you are getting all the nutrients you need without packing on too many calories. Focus on including a lot of different nutrient-dense foods and skip all the "low fat" and "diet" versions of foods. In order to make a food low fat, manufactures usually add a lot of extra sugar to make up for the loss in flavor. But sugar (*not* fat) is one of the leading causes of weight gain.

Diet foods often contain artificial and heavily processed ingredients (like hydrogenated fats and artificial sweeteners). These artificial ingredients are things your body has no idea how to break down and use so, instead of digesting them, it simply stores them as fat until it can figure out what to do with them. Basically, "diet" soda and other "diet" foods are actually causing you to gain more weight. Your best option is to stick to natural, whole foods—foods with ingredients that you can identify. If there's a long list of unpronounceable ingredients, put it back on the shelf and move on.

Once you have created your healthy menu for the week, gather all your ingredients and spend the afternoon cooking. When you cook in bulk and cook all at once, you'll spend less total time cooking than you would if you prepared each meal separately throughout the week. Your breakfasts may be simple enough that you can just prepare them every morning instead of making them all at once and storing them. But your lunches and dinners probably need to be prepared in advance so that you can save time during the week without sacrificing your goal of losing weight or your health. You can make your weekly cooking day a fun family activity. Teach your children the same healthy habits that you are trying to adopt so they grow up with the right attitudes and skills toward food to live long, healthy, happy lives.

Everyday Habit #4

Cut This Out & Lose Weight FASTER Than Before!

Of all the meals of the day, your dinner should take the longest to digest. You want foods that are slow to break down so that your stomach is too busy digesting in the evening to feel cravings. What this means is that you want a lot of protein and fat without as many simple carbohydrates. Of all the kinds of foods out there, carbohydrates digest the fastest. This leads to sharp spikes in your blood glucose levels followed by equally sharp drops. This is exactly what causes cravings—especially cravings for sweets.

When your body experiences sudden and fast drops in blood glucose, it begins to panic and look for more carbohydrates to quickly restore your glucose levels. So try to cut out carbohydrates from your dinner. At the very least, you need to cut out simple carbohydrates. Simple carbohydrates are sugars, refined flours, and starchy foods (potatoes, sticky rice, etc.) A good way to identify and eliminate simple carbohydrates is to remember to avoid white foods: white bread, refined white sugar, potatoes, and so on.

Of course, there are some white foods that don't fit on this list (milk, cauliflower, etc.) but in general, this is how you can safely avoid simple carbohydrates. Complex carbohydrates are the ones that take more time for your body to digest like high fiber foods and vegetables. They still digest more quickly than proteins and fats but it's slow enough (and adds enough nutrition to your diet) that you don't need to avoid them.

The reason you want to cut down the carbohydrates at dinner is because you don't need the energy boost they offer when you're just going to be relaxing and then going to bed. Instead, you want your dinner to be a meal that digests slowly and keeps your stomach busy all night so that you are less likely to run to the kitchen for a late-night snack before bed.

Action Plan

Make protein and fat the key parts of your dinner without going over your calorie budget by slightly decreasing the amount of protein and fat you eat for breakfast and lunch. For example, to get your 50 grams of protein, eat 12 grams for breakfast, 13 grams for lunch, and 25 grams for dinner. To get the 30 grams of fat, you can eat 5 grams at breakfast, 5 grams at lunch and 20 grams at dinner. Between 25 grams of protein and 20 grams of fat, your dinner is going to easily keep you full through the night.

At the same time that you are increase the protein and fat, decrease the carbohydrates. You need 30 grams of fiber (which comes exclusively from complex carbohydrate foods). To get this, eat 10 grams for breakfast, 15 grams for lunch and 5 grams at dinner. The other benefit of making your breakfast and lunch high in complex carbohydrates while your dinner is high in protein and fat is that the carbohydrates give you a faster boost to your glucose levels (i.e. - your energy). That means that during the day, when you need to have the most energy, your meals are giving you the perfect balance of fast-acting energy and stable, sustained energy.

Come dinner when it's time to relax and slow down, you'll have a slow-digesting meal that will help keep you from getting late night cravings and avoid those extra, after dinner snacks. Avoid simple carbohydrates throughout the day, every day. The only sugar that you should be getting is the small amount that comes from fruits. Cut out *all* foods that have added sugar. If you have a serious sweet tooth, this will be difficult at first. But trust me, after a few weeks of sticking to the no-added sugar rule, it will get easier and easier. Soon, you'll be able to enjoy the natural sweetness of fruits and even start disliking excessively sugary foods.

Everyday Habit #5

Make Sleep a Priority

Your first thought might be: how can sleep possibly help me lose weight? You burn the *least* amount of calories while sleeping. Well, this chapter will explain the very important role that sleeps plays in weight loss and your overall health. It won't take a lot of convincing to tell you that you need to get a good night's sleep every night. You probably already know the difference between how you feel after a night of quality sleep in comparison to a night of too little sleep. But it does more than just make you feel more alert and energized in the morning.

Here are some of the other reasons that sleep is so essential:

1. **Lack of sleep causes cravings:** when you wake up feeling tired and unenergetic, you usually reach for a big cup of coffee and a sugary treat to give you the boost you need. If you had gotten a good night sleep, you would wake up feeling naturally energized and alert. Instead of desperately going for a fast-sugary boost, you could prepare and eat a healthy, balanced breakfast.

2. **Lack of sleep slows metabolism:** just as you lack energy in the morning after a bad night of restless sleep, so does your metabolism. Your digestive system is triggered by the same hormones that regulate your sleep cycle. The hormone that tells your brain to feel alert also tells your metabolism to rev up and start producing energy. Without enough sleep, you don't get these wake-up hormones (because your body literally doesn't want you to wake up yet) which means your metabolism doesn't get the signal to start working.

3. **Sleep helps you avoid late night snacking:** the logic is simple enough. If you are asleep, you can't eat (well, unless you are a sleep-eater). So instead of staying up until 3am surfing on the internet, get to bed early enough (at least 6 or 7 hours before you plan to wake up) to make sure that you get a full night of sleep and avoid the midnight munchies.

4. **Sleep helps you burn fat:** studies show that sleep helps your body burn fat. Two people who eat the exact same low-calorie diet will not burn the same amount of fat if they don't get the same amount of sleep. For example, in one study, people ate the same number of calories but one group slept

8.5 hours per night while the other group slept just 5.5 hours per night. By the end of the study, both groups had lost an average of 6.5 pounds. But when they measured where those pounds came from, the results were surprising. For the group that slept 5.5 hours per night, only 25% of those pounds were from fat. For the group that got a full night of sleep, however, more than 50% of the pounds lost were fat.

5. **Sleep helps you eat less calories:** not only does it help you stop snacking late at night but it helps you naturally lower the number of calories you eat during the day. Many studies have been done on this subject and they have found that people who get a full night of sleep eat an average of 700 fewer calories per day than people who don't get enough sleep. That is a truly significant amount. 700 fewer calories per day could translate to up to 2 pounds of weight loss per week!

Action Plan

Now that you know how important sleep is and how it can help you with your weight loss and health goals, it's time to learn how you can make sure that you sleep better and get the sleep that you need. The first step is to stop doing things that are hurting your ability to fall asleep and sleep well.

Here are some of the things that you need to stop doing:

1. **Stop looking at screens**: the backlight that comes out of your computer screen, phone screen, tablet screen, or television screen is a similar frequency as the light that comes from the sun. Because your body is programmed to respond to sunlight as a signal that it's time to be awake and alert, looking at screens (which emit light similar to sunlight) can damage your body's natural sleep and wake cycle. You don't have to give up technology altogether. But you do need

to put it away and stop using it 4 hours before you plan to go to sleep.

2. **Stop eating before bed**: eating right before bed so that you have a bloated, full stomach will make it more difficult for you to fall asleep because your body is too busy digesting to fall into the relaxed mental state you should be in so that you can get some quality shut eye. You don't need to go to bed hungry but avoid eating anything at least 1 hour before bed. This means avoiding late night dinners and especially late-night snacks. Your body needs some time to get through the initial stages of digestion before you try to fall asleep.

3. **Stop having cold feet**: no, this doesn't mean you need to resolve any commitment issues you might have, it just means you need to put on a pair of socks. As your body starts to relax, your circulation slows down and the first parts to suffer are your feet because they are furthest from your heart. In order for your body to get relaxed, it needs to feel warm and cozy. So slip on a pair of socks if it's particularly cold.

4. **Stop stressing**: this one is definitely easier said than done. But it is worth making the effort. If you're worried about something that is going to happen tomorrow or in the future (or your worried about the consequences of something that did happen), try to think through and find a solution during the day. When you are trying to fall asleep, stress and worrying are just going to keep you tossing and turning. So do your best to focus on positive thoughts before bed, knowing that if you wake up feeling refreshed and energized, you have a far better chance of finding a solution than if you are groggy and unable to be fully alert. If all your best efforts fail and you still find yourself worrying about a problem at night, at least try to focus on thinking about possible

solutions rather than just focusing on the negatives and the worst-case scenario.

5. **Stop working in bed**: you need to make sure that your bed is for sleep (and maybe also for making new family members!). Don't bring your laptop into bed to study, work, or chat with friends. Your bed is not chair or table. Your bedroom is not a living room. You want your body to get the clear message that when you are in bed that means it is time to sleep. If you do anything else in bed, this message won't be clear.

In addition to stopping these bad bedtime habits, you should set up some healthy bedtime habits that will help you fall asleep more easily and get better quality sleep:

1. **Establish a bedtime routine**: you need to have a stable routine that you go through every night before bed. Do the same things in the same order every night. This repetition helps your body realize what's going on. If you always brush your teeth, wash your face, and put on pajamas (in that order) before laying down in bed, your body will already know as soon as the toothbrush hits your teeth that it's time to sleep. This will help you fall asleep more quickly when you finally lay down. Having this routine also means not doing these things any other time of day (except for brushing your teeth, please brush your teeth more than once a day!). For example, don't wear pajamas during the daytime. You can have other comfy clothes for a day of relaxing at home but don't wear the same things you wear to bed.

2. **Keep the room cold**: studies have shown that a cold room helps you sleep better than a warm room. This doesn't mean it needs to be freezing but does need to be cooler than usual. Your body naturally lowers its temperature while you are sleeping. When the temperature of your room is closer to the

temperature that your body is trying to lower to, it will help you get to sleep faster. Normally, it is advised to keep the thermostat somewhere between 65- and 72-degrees Fahrenheit. But some people feel more comfortable in lower temperatures (or higher temperatures). A good rule of thumb is to lower the temperature about 5 degrees from wherever you like to set it during the day.

3. **Go to bed and wake up at the same time**: this is important for the same reasons that having a steady bedtime routine is important. By going to bed at the same time every single night, you are allowing your body to establish a stable biorhythm. It can regulate your hormone cycles so that you get a surge of the hormones that help you wake up in the morning and a surge of the hormones that help you sleep when you are trying to go to sleep. When you go to bed and wake up at the same time every day, your body learns when to release which hormones. So avoid pulling any all-nighters and try to wake up at the same time each morning (even if it's a weekend and you could sleep in). You can't "make up" for lost sleep on the weekends, anyway. That's not how your body works. So it's more important to keep a stable sleep schedule than to keep changing your bedtime and your wake up time.

4. **Read a book**: Make sure it's made of paper or it's on an eReader that uses the ink technology to look like real paper instead of having backlight coming out of the screen. As mentioned above, you want to avoid screens before bed. If you have trouble keeping your racing thoughts at bay, a book can help distract your mind and make you feel relaxed. Get a small book light that you can attach to the book so you can turn off all the other lights and keep the room dark. The darkness will help your body get sleepy and the act of reading will help relax your mind and get it ready for sleep.

Everyday Habit #6

Cut the Caffeine

A cup of coffee in the morning is a great way to jumpstart your day. The caffeine wakes you up and speeds up your metabolism. If you drink it without milk or sugar, it is also the ideal zero calorie treat. But beyond 1 or 2 cups in the morning, you should be careful about how much caffeine you consume in a day. Too much caffeine raises blood pressure, increases anxiety, and can keep you awake at night when you are trying to go to sleep. Coffee isn't the only source of caffeine. It is also found in soda, tea, chocolate, and even certain pain medications (because it also helps relieve headaches). So, watch what you eat and drink throughout the day and try to avoid consuming any kind of caffeine at least 4 hours before you plan to go to sleep at night.

Caffeine is a stimulant, which means it keeps your brain awake and alert even when your body is exhausted and ready to call it a day. Because you need a good, full night of rest every night in order to promote health and weight loss, consuming caffeine to close to your bedtime is going to cause you to gain weight. In addition to the negative effects of drinking more than 1 or 2 cups of coffee per day, there are a host of other negative health effects to drinking other caffeinated beverages.

The biggest offender is, by far, soda. Regular soda is bad and diet soda is even worse. Often, soda is loaded with corn syrup or, in the case of diet soda, artificial sweeteners like aspartame. Your body cannot recognize either of these ingredients and doesn't know how to break them down. So, for lack of any other option, it just stores them as fat. If you drink soda or consume a lot of foods and beverages that have either corn syrup or an artificial sweetener, this is, undoubtedly, a major factor in any excess weight you have gained. As soon as you cut these out of your diet, you will notice significant weight loss. Sodas (whether diet or not) are also very high in sodium. Diets that are high in sodium cause high blood pressure, dehydration, and weight gain. If you consume too much sodium, your body will start to retain a lot of water which means you'll bloat up with a lot of water weight.

Excess sodium, especially when you are already not drinking enough water every day, also leads to dehydration. Dehydration causes weight gain, slowed metabolism, as well as many other serious health problems. So, next time you are feeling thirsty, soda is the absolute last thing you should drink. Rather than quenching your thirst, soda is actually making you *thirstier*.

Too much caffeine can also lead to dehydration because, in addition to being a stimulant, caffeine is also a diuretic. Diuretics are things that cause you to get rid of more fluid than they add. In the simplest terms, they make you urinate a lot. You end up expelling more fluids from urination than you took in from drinking the caffeinated beverage. If you don't drink enough water to replace those lost fluids, you will become dehydrated which is extremely unhealthy and also causes weight gain. So, cut your total caffeine intake to about 200 milligrams per day (or 2 coffee mugs worth of coffee). Cut soda out of your diet entirely.

Action Plan

If you drink coffee in the morning, start decreasing the amount of milk or sugar that you add—if you add any. Drinking black coffee will give you a stronger effect from the beginning and help you drink less in total. You simply cannot chug a whole cup of hot black coffee. Without milk to cool it down and sugar to dampen the flavor, you'll be forced to sip slowly and enjoy it at a relaxed pace. Start cutting out any other caffeine you normally drink after your morning coffee and completely cut out caffeinated beverages 4 hours before you plan to go to sleep.

In the evenings, drink herbal teas that are naturally caffeine free to replace your normal coffee, soda, or black tea. Mint tea is an especially good option because it is naturally caffeine free and the mint will even help you fight cravings. Remember to drink more water throughout the day as well in order to make sure you are fully hydrated. If you make an effort to stay hydrated throughout the day, you will reduce feelings of fatigue and maintain full alertness. This means you won't feel the need to get those regular doses of caffeine to keep you going through the day. You need at least 2 liters of water every day. You can start your day off better by drinking a glass of water with your coffee in the morning. Water in the morning will help wake up your metabolism.

Since coffee is already a metabolism booster, drinking a glass of water with your coffee will act as a double strength boost so you can be sure there is nothing sluggish about your metabolism even if you might still be feeling a little tired in the morning. As for soda, you should cut this out entirely. If you are a regular soda drinking, this will be more challenging. Soda can be a genuine addiction but it is absolutely worth the struggle. Even after 1 week of being soda free, you will already notice amazing changes. You'll lose weight, you'll feel more clear-headed and focused, you'll feel more energetic throughout the day rather than experiencing those peaks and crashes of energy that normally come with soda. The list of benefits you'll get from not drinking soda could fill up a book of their own.

If your soda habit is really serious and you actually experience withdrawal-like symptoms, here are a few tips to help you kick the habit:

- **Drink a soda substitute**: buy plain carbonated water and mix it with juice (no sugar added). Alternatively, you can mix it with fresh fruits. Berries are an especially delicious option. It won't be a perfect imitation of soda because it is caffeine free, sodium free, and without any added sugar. However, it has that carbonated feel that you look for in a can of soda and it will have some sweetness from the juice or fruit that you add. So it allows you to sort of go through the motions of drinking soda and get the experience without getting the added weight and other health problems.

- **Go cold turkey**: with some things, you can cut them out gradually. Soda is not one of those things. It is better to go cold turkey. This might sound painful at first but it will make the process of breaking the habits go much more quickly. So decide today to stop drinking soda and give it up entirely. Don't make excuses.

- **Throw out all the soda in your house**: if there is soda in your house, you are going to drink it. That's all there is to it. It's like a smoker who keeps a pack of cigarettes in her purse and says, "I'm not going to smoke them. I'm just hanging on to them." If your children or partner also drink soda, tell them they are quitting the habit too. It is better for their health. Plus, making sure that nobody else has soda in the house will help you stay away from the stuff yourself. Your kids might get mad at you but let them get mad. They will thank you later when they grow up without diabetes, obesity, or any other health problem that soda causes.

- **Take it one day at a time**: don't try to focus on how hard it is going to be to never drink soda again. First of all, it is not going to be that hard. After the first 30 days, you'll already find it easier to go without it. Give it another 30 days after that and you'll already find yourself going a whole week without ever even thinking about it. Secondly, worrying about the road ahead will only make it more difficult to navigate the road right in front of you. Track your progress and take pride in every single day that you go without soda. Just focus on getting through the next 24 hours. When you've gotten through that, focus on getting through the next 24 hours.

- **Don't beat yourself up**: when you first try to kick the soda habit, you are going to slip up. You're going to have cravings you simply cannot resist. Fight these cravings with everything you've got. But when you cave in and have a soda, don't feel like it was all a waste of your effort. And don't feel like you are too weak to get through this. You have still come a long way and you are still further than you were when you started. Most importantly, you can still get right back up and keep going. Think of it this way: if you normally drink about 2 sodas every day and after doing a 30 day soda free challenge, you slipped up 5 times, that would still be 50 sodas that you *didn't* drink! That is fantastic progress. The next 30 days will be that much easier because of that accomplishment. Change is not a switch that you flip. It is a journey that you have to take. If you feel weak now, remember that nobody is strong enough to make it to the end right when they start. You gather the strength along the way, with each step that you take, each mistake that you make, and each obstacle that you overcome.

So kick your soda habit, keep your coffee for the morning, and replace evening caffeine with herbal teas or carbonated water with fruits. This sounds like a lot for one habit but the results are well worth the effort.

Everyday Habit #7

Avoid Alcohol & Tobacco

Alcohol and tobacco should be kept to a minimum no matter whom you are or what you are trying to accomplish. In excess, these two can cause extremely serious health problems from liver failure to lung cancer. So, try to save them for special occasions only and even then, only in moderation. Beyond the many health problems that are associated with alcohol and tobacco (you probably have already heard and read plenty about each of them), they can also contribute to weight gain.

Let's start with tobacco. The nicotine in tobacco acts as a stimulant. That is, it keeps you awake and alert. In excess, this can cause heightened anxiety and stress (which smokers usually try to fight by smoking more, resulting in even worse anxiety and stress). If you smoke within 1 to 2 hours of going to bed, you will have a more difficult time falling asleep because your brain is still simulated and alert from the nicotine. As you already know by now, a lack of quality sleep can have serious consequences on your health and your weight. So if you are a smoker and don't have any intention of quitting, you should, at the very least, avoid smoking 1 hour before you plan to go to sleep. You should actually also consider quitting entirely but that is a topic for another book. Try to cut your overall total down to 10 cigarettes per day in order to minimize the anxiety and stress that smoking causes.

Now let's take a look at the weight gain effects of alcohol. First of all, alcoholic drinks are deceptively high in calories, especially if you are partial to those fancy, sugary cocktails. If you've ever heard someone mention "beer bellies", you should know that they are a real thing. To give you an idea: one margarita has 153 calories, 12 ounces of beer averages about 150 to 200 calories, and a single shot of tequila will pack 96 calories. That means a night of drinking could end up adding more calories than you ate the entire day! Opting for the low calorie or light options isn't going to help you much, either. Like caffeine, alcohol is also a diuretic, causing you to expel more water than you take in from drinking it. It is a more powerful diuretic than caffeine, too. This is one of the main reasons you get a hangover after a night of drinking. An 8-oz. alcoholic beverage will cause you to expel about 33 oz. of water! So, if you aren't drinking water by the gallon as you drink alcohol, you are on the road to severe dehydration.

As you already know, chronic dehydration is one of the factors that contribute to weight gain. One night of drinking can set you back pretty far. So far, alcohol packs on a ridiculous amount of calories and causes severe dehydration. But alcohol leads to weight gain in another, less well-known way as well. When you consume alcohol, your body switches gears. It is not possible for your body to store any excess alcohol as fat so it has to burn up all the calories as they come in. This means that the fat burning process that your body typically goes through during the entire day comes to a complete stop. It even stops metabolizing the other things in your stomach because it is entirely focused on dealing with the alcohol. So, alcohol is a fat building offender on 3 fronts: it adds calories, it dehydrates you, and it completely stops your body from burning fat.

Action Plan

If you are planning to go out drinking, drink a tall glass of water between each alcoholic beverage you have. This will not only help replace some of the lost water but will also slow down your drinking and help you drink less.

When you get home, chug a liter of water before bed. You can also try to get a jump-start by drinking more than your usual 2 liters during the day. Try to drink double the amount of water before you start, continue to drink water as you drink alcohol, and end the night with a lot of water. This will help prevent dehydration but it won't get rid of the calories. For those, you'll have to get in some serious dancing during the night!

If you aren't going out to drink but you would like to have some wine or beer at home, drink it with dinner and keep it down to 1 or 2 glasses. Your body needs 1 hour to fully metabolize 1 portion of alcohol. For reference, 1 portion is equal to a 5-oz. glass of wine, a

12-oz. bottle of beer, or a 1.5 oz. shot of hard liquor. This means you shouldn't drink too close to bed time because you want to give your body the full amount of time it needs to metabolize the alcohol before you go to sleep. While you may think that alcohol helps you sleep, this is only partially true. It does help you fall asleep more quickly but it prevents your body from going to REM sleep (the most restful kind of sleep). So, your overall quality of sleep is poorer if you have alcohol in your system.

With that in mind, it is okay to have that glass or two of wine with your dinner but make sure you have dinner early enough that you have enough hours left before bed to fully metabolize the alcohol. During those hours that you are metabolizing, drink enough water to replace the total amount of fluid lost from alcohol. For every ounce of alcohol you drank, you need to drink 4 ounces of water.

As for smoking: don't have a cigarette within one hour before you plan to go to bed and try to keep your daily total down to 10 cigarettes. This will help reduce the impact smoking has on your sleep quality and lower your overall stress levels throughout the day.

Everyday Habit #8

This Will STOP Evening Food Cravings

If you've already eaten dinner and you still have the urge to munch on something, it is mostly likely because your dinner wasn't satisfying enough. Later on in this book, you'll learn more about how to make a satisfying dinner that will help stop cravings before they even start. But, if a satisfying, balanced dinner still can't kill the cravings, try brushing your teeth. This probably sounds a little odd. But it actually works. After brushing your teeth, you won't want to eat anything because the minty flavor won't mix well with food.

Toothpaste and barbecue flavored chips? No, thank you. Plus, who wants to ruin freshly cleaned teeth with junk food? You actually need to wait 30 minutes after brushing your teeth to eat anyway because you need to give the enamel coating on your teeth time to harden again. Brushing your teeth is also effective because the mint in the toothpaste acts as a craving-fighter. Mint is often used to help stave off strong cravings and control appetite.

Action Plan

Try brushing your teeth right after dinner so that you will be less likely to snack throughout the night. Alternatively, you can wait about an hour after dinner or whenever the cravings really start to kick in. To be most effective, you should do it before the cravings truly start. Try to estimate about how long after dinner you get the urge to start snacking and brush your teeth about 5 to 10 minutes before that time.

Everyday Habit #9

Don't Confuse Thirst for Hunger

Recent studies show that as much as 75% of Americans may be suffering from chronic dehydration. That figure is staggering. That means that 3 out of every 4 people in the United States are chronically dehydrated! Now, your first thought might be, "okay, that is definitely shocking but what exactly does that have to do with losing weight?" The answer is: everything.

Chronic dehydration causes our bodies to lose the ability to recognize when we are thirsty (which leads to further dehydration). In fact, our thirst receptors are so low that we often confuse thirst for hunger. For example, if you've ever started to feel a little weak or gotten a headache and thought, "oh, I should probably eat something", you are probably wrong. Most of the time, these symptoms are signs that your body needs water—no, not soda, not sugary juice, not coffee. It needs water.

Without water, your body simply cannot function. Your body is 60% water. You need it to lubricate your brain, your muscles, your digestive system, and literally everything else. If you are not drinking at least 2 liters of water per day, you are not drinking enough water. Chronic dehydration can actually lead to weight gain in addition to a dizzying list of other problems. It leads to digestive disorders, bladder problems, kidney problems, constipation, fatigue and a lot of other health issues that end up causing you to store more fat in the body instead of efficiently burning it off as energy.

Being dehydrated can also lead to irresistible cravings for sugary foods. This is because dehydration means your body doesn't have the water it needs to release glycogen, which is needed to stabilize the glucose levels in your blood. Blood glucose is what your body uses as energy. When your glucose levels are low, you start craving sweets because sugar can be turned into glucose quickly. If you're dehydrated, you don't actually need to rely on sugar, you just need to drink water so that you can use the energy stores you already have in you.

Water has so many amazing benefits for weight loss, health, and appearance that it's amazing we aren't all guzzling it down on a regular basis.

Here are a few of the benefits of staying thoroughly hydrated:

- **Decrease calories**: water is a zero-calorie method to fighting cravings. As mentioned earlier, most people confuse the signs of dehydration with the signs of hunger and end up eating when a glass of water would actually be more satisfying for your body.

- **Boost metabolism**: water in your body is like oil in your car's engine. It keeps things running smoothly and that includes your digestive system. Your stomach is able to breakdown nutrients more easily and your body can transport those nutrients to the rest of your body more quickly.

- **Clears skin**: drinking enough water helps prevent your pores from getting clogged and reduces the appearance of wrinkles by increasing skin elasticity. This means you'll have smoother, less pimply skin without having to follow some elaborate skin care routine.

- **Improve focus and alertness**: dehydration slows the brain down along with the rest of the body. Some studies have shown that a glass of water could actually be more effective than a cup of coffee when it comes to making you feel more alert, awake, and ready to concentrate on the task at hand.

- **Prevents constipation**: as mentioned earlier, staying hydrated helps to keep things running smoothly. In fact, one of the leading causes of constipation is dehydration. So to avoid getting backed up, make sure you are drinking enough water every day.

Action Plan

The best way to make sure you are hydrated is pretty simple: drink water. And when I say drink water, I really mean water, not juice or coffee and *especially* not soda. Cut down on the amount of beverages you buy so that when you are at home, your only real option for drinking is water. You might think water is plain and boring but it is a completely nonnegotiable necessity. You need to drink 2 liters of water every single day. Get a water bottle (preferably metal or glass) and figure out how many times you need to refill to make your 2-liter requirement. For example, if you've got a 1-liter bottle, you'll only need to drink 2 full bottles. Keep this water bottle with you and drink regularly throughout the day. When you are feeling a little sleepy, drink water. When you are starting to feel a craving for snacks come on, drink water.

In addition to drinking water all throughout the day, you should drink water with every meal. Don't eat without having some water to wash it down. You can even use water to help slow your pace which, as you have already learned, is another healthy weight loss habit you should practice. Take a sip of water after swallowing each bite to help you eat fewer total calories and help your digestive system break down the food more easily.

Everyday Habit #10

The CURE to Night Binges Fits in Your Pocket!

One of the reasons we enjoy snacking at night so much is because it keeps our body busy while we are watching TV. Even if you aren't actually hungry, you just enjoy chewing while you watch your favorite show. To get the satisfaction of chewing and help fight cravings, you can try chewing sugarless mint gum. The mint (as you learned earlier in this book) will help fight your cravings while the act of chewing will keep you busy as you watch TV or surf the internet.

Action Plan

When you get the urge to snack after dinner, try chewing a piece of sugarless mint gum instead. Buy a bulk package of it and keep it at home so that you'll always have gum as an option to avoid snacking. It's a good way to trick yourself and avoid packing on calories.

Everyday Habit #11

Take an After-Dinner Walk

As you'll learn in the next chapter, watching TV is a major contributor to weight gain. Countless studies have been done on the links between TV and obesity and what they have found is surprising (you'll get the specific numbers in the next chapter). Not only is it a sedentary activity that doesn't help you burn off calories, it is a major trigger for snacking. If you have trouble avoiding those snacks after dinner, try going for a walk.

Walks burn calories, reduce cravings, decrease stress, and get you out of the house so you don't spend as much time sitting around. It can also boost your metabolism in a few different ways. For one, exercise triggers your metabolism and revs it up into a higher gear. But walking also decreases stress. You might remember from the first chapter (about eating slowly and enjoying your food) about how stress causes your metabolism to slow down. It redirects the calories to be stored as fat.

So, a nice walk after dinner can really get your metabolism going to help you burn off extra calories. A brisk 30-minute walk will burn around 150 calories. At the same time, you'll be out of the house and away from the temptation to start munching. So, add the calories you burned to the number of calories you *didn't* eat and you'll really start to see some change.

There are also a lot of other benefits to walking that go beyond weight loss:

- **Heart health**: daily walks can reduce your bad cholesterol and increase your good cholesterol. It also helps keep blood pressure under control. That same brisk 30-minute walk that's burning 150 calories for you will also reduce your risk for heart disease and stroke by 27%!

- **Prevent disease**: walking can also decrease your risk for type 2 diabetes, certain cancers, and even asthma attacks. In fact, one study showed that people who made a daily habit of walking had a 20% lower risk of getting breast cancer, colon cancer, and cancer of the uterus. So, every woman should make a point to walk at least 30 minutes per day.

- **Increase muscle mass**: walking is a form of exercise so it helps you build muscle. You won't become an international bodybuilding champion but you'll see some welcome muscle tone in your legs and stomach. Plus, the more muscle you have, the more calories you burn (because muscles need more calories to operate than fat). So, this is yet another weight loss benefit you can get from taking an after-dinner walk.

- **Avoid dementia**: as you age, there are a whole range of new diseases you'll have to start worrying about. About 1 in every 14 people over the age of 65 already has dementia. That jumps to 1 in every 6 people for people over 80. However, walking keeps your brain healthy and strong. Long-term studies have shown that people who take walks every day were 40% less likely to show signs of dementia when they got older. This is because walking prevents brain shrinkage, which tends to happen as you age.

- **Maintain strong bones**: in addition to dementia, you'll also have to start thinking about osteoporosis when you hit your golden years. As you age, your bone density begins to decrease. This is especially the case if you snack on a lot of calcium-poor junk food and don't get any exercise. So, in addition to getting more calcium in your diet, you should start walking daily to keep your bones strong and prevent osteoporosis in old age.

- **Boost your energy**: if you're feeling lazy or lack motivation, then forcing yourself to go for a walk can give you that surge of energy you need to power through a late-night project or even just feel better in general. It improves your circulation, increases your oxygen supply and keeps you feeling alert. It'll help stretch out stiff joints and reduce muscle pain. So, if you've been sitting all day, a walk is the perfect thing to get rid of that aching, sluggish feeling you get from sitting around for too long.

- **Improve your mood**: moderate exercise of all kinds (and this includes walking) releases neurotransmitters in your brain that allow you to feel pleasure. This can decrease depression, anxiety, and stress.

  As you already learned, stress slows the metabolism down and pleasure speeds it up. So not only will you feel better, you'll be helping your metabolism out as well! Who knew just being happy could help you lose weight?

After reading about all these benefits, you're probably ready to start making walking part of your evening routine. Here are a few tips to help you stick with it.

Action Plan

Don't accept excuses. As soon as you clear the table after dinner, put on your walking shoes and get outside. You might be feeling lazy while you're inside the house but as soon as you get out of the front door and you take your first breath of cool, evening air, you'll be ready to go. So just skip all the excuses and put on those shoes already!

If you've got a family, have them join you. An evening walk is a great family activity no matter what age your kids are. Even if you've got an infant, pushing the stroller will just lead to more calories burned! Plus, if your little one has a tough time falling asleep, a ride in the stroller will usually help them pass right out. You'll be helping yourself lose weight and instilling the right habits in your children for when they get older.

If you've got a pet, going for a walk will be even more fun (assuming your pet is not a goldfish, that is). Your dog's motivation and excitement about going for a walk will help you get motivated yourself. After a few days of nightly walks, your dog will push you to stick with the habit even on the evenings when you're having doubts. And how can you say no to that adorable puppy face? If you don't have pet, consider getting one! Not only will they get you up and walking, they decrease stress, which, as you know, is a great boost to your weight loss efforts.

Whether you are walking alone or walking with family, the trick is to just do it. Don't do any other activity after dinner before you have taken your walk. It should just become an automatic part of dinnertime. You haven't finished until you've gotten back from your walk. As soon as you turn on the TV or start surfing the Internet, it's going to be a lot harder to motivate yourself to get out the door. So, walk first, be lazy later.

The bottom line is you just need to start walking! 30 minutes after dinner of walking is all it takes to get the full range of benefits that walking has to offer. That's 30 minutes of getting exercise, boosting your metabolism, decreasing stress, decreasing disease, burning calories, and countless other things. No TV show, no matter how good, can offer you those kinds of benefits!

Everyday Habit #12

Turn off the T.V.

If you have ever in your life eaten food purely out of boredom, then you already know the dangers of letting your mind or body get bored. While the television might seem like a cure for boredom, it's more of a distraction from the bored feeling. It doesn't stimulate your mind or get your body moving. It just flashes some nice colors and sounds at you so you don't have to think about boredom.

To kill boredom, you need activities that actually require some thinking or physical action—or both! One of the reasons snacking goes so well with watching TV is that your body is just desperate for something to do instead of just sitting there. You need to add more stimulating activities to your evening schedule to keep your mind off that package of string cheese in the fridge that's calling your name. The average American watches 5 hours of television every day. This fact alone is enough to decide that you should cut down on the amount of television. You could use that time to do so many other enjoyable things. But if you combine that with the fact the average personal also eats between 100 and 300 calories during 1 hour of watching television, the numbers become even more shocking. Think of how much weight you could lose just by cutting out one hour of TV per day? That would be 7 hours less per week, which could work out to as much as 2,100 fewer calories per week depending on how much you snack while in front of the TV. If you cut TV out entirely, and replace it with something healthy, such as walking, you could flip your calories in/out balance for the entire week by up to 5,000 calories! The numbers are staggering. So, it's worth dropping your television time and finding a better way to relax when you get home from work in the evening.

Action Plan

Try reading a book. It's got characters, plots, and drama just like your TV shows but it requires more brain activity because you have to actively read the words on the page and then interpret the meaning of the words and the sentence as a whole. Of course, you don't consciously think about interpreting the meaning but your brain is doing it. The reason it doesn't do the same thing when you've got the TV on is because the images on the screen already do half the work for you. You don't have to imagine what the characters look like, how they said something, what their voice might look like, or even what the background setting looks like when it's all already there on the screen. When your brain is busy using imagination, it's going to spend less time imagining the snacks in your kitchen.

If you're not a huge fan of reading (with the exception of this book, at least), my first suggestion is to give it another chance. There are so many books out there that you are bound to find something that sparks your interest. And in this age of eBooks, you have easy access to millions of books. But if you are still reluctant to choose a book over the TV, try other activities. Get crafty by making your own jewelry, soaps, clothes, or literally anything else. Learn a new language or practice a new skill. Have a game night with the family or take up gardening. Start painting or drawing.

In fact, here are dozens of things that you can do instead of snacking to take your mind off the munchies:

- Light some scented candles and take a long, hot bat
- Invite your partner into the tub with you!

- Organize your home office or your closet
- Try knitting or crocheting
- Treat yourself to a spa evening: facials, manicures, the whole nine yards
- Put on your favorite music and dance
- Have an impromptu dance party with the whole family!
- Invite your friends while you're at it!
- Start keeping a journal and write in it
- Go through old pictures and reminisce
- Annoy your pets
- Water your plants (alternatively: buy some plants. Then water them)
- Get rid of clothes you don't want
- Go shopping to replace the clothes you got rid of
- Learn to play an instrument
- Call a friend or relative to chat
- Play solitaire (like, with actual cards)
- Build a house out of cards (then knock it over when you get frustrated with them)
- Plan a weekend trip for the family (or a weekend getaway with your friends)
- Find creative new uses for things in your house
- Make sock monkeys with the kids
- Actually try one of those cool ideas you saw on the internet
- Do something that you have been procrastinating on for too long

There are hundreds of things you can do instead of watch TV. This doesn't mean you have to throw out your television. Just only watch it when you have a specific show you enjoy watching. Then, turn it off when it's over and do something else. If you ever catch yourself flipping through the channels to see what's on, that's the sign it's time to turn it off and do something else. Once you get into the habit of doing other things aside from watching TV, not only will you keep yourself distracted from snacking, you'll also free up a lot of time to do activities that are way more rewarding. You're going to wonder why you ever wasted so much time flipping through channels to look for something that was at least moderately entertaining. There's a whole wide world out there (or even a whole wide house out there) that's waiting for you to explore its opportunities. You'll be able to have more quality time with your loved ones and build lasting memories. When you do decide to turn on the TV, do something else instead of snacking. For example, watching TV can be the perfect time to power through some crunches or if your living room is big enough, put a treadmill in there and go for a run while watching your favorite show.

Everyday Habit #13

Curb Cravings with Nutrition (Part I)

The battle against between meal cravings begins with nutrition. If you get all the nutrients you need from your 3 main meals of the day, your body simply won't have any need to crave snacks in between. Your cravings are not some mysterious part of your subconscious mind; it's a simple matter of your body feeling like it doesn't have enough. Of course, there is some psychology to it. Some people practice "emotional eating." That is, they eat in order to avoid dealing with negative emotions. This is where the cliché of eating a big tub of ice cream after a breakup comes from. But the primary factor in cravings is poor nutrition so if you eat a healthy diet, you won't have as many between meal cravings and the cravings you do have will start to be for healthier foods rather than junk and sweets. So in part I, we are going to focus on fiber.

Fiber is a powerful tool against weight loss. It helps you feel fuller and it is a huge boost to your metabolism. In fact, if you ate absolutely no fiber, you wouldn't be able to digest food. Your body needs fiber in order to push the food through your whole system and finally expel it. Because fiber takes more time to break down than sugars and other junk foods, it keeps you feeling full and satisfied for a lot longer and adds a lot less calories. It also stabilizes your glucose levels because it acts as a shield that slows your body's absorption of glucose. So it stabilizes the rate at which your body gets the energy from your food instead of just sending it all as one big burst at the beginning. This means you avoid the peak and crash cycle that comes with a high sugar diet.

Fiber also helps control your appetite because, although it is low in calories, it is a really bulky form of nutrition. It takes up a lot of space in the stomach and moves slowly throughout your digestive system so you end up feeling full after eating less. Fiber is what gives vegetables their crispy texture and whole grain breads their full-bodied flavor. Fiber is why a spoonful of peanut butter feels a lot more satisfying and filling than a spoonful of jelly. It is also what helps you digest and use the other nutrients in your food. Studies have shown that fiber improves your body's ability to absorb minerals like calcium, zinc, and magnesium. So, if you take a daily supplement, make sure you eat a high fiber meal with it so you can make sure your body absorbs as much as possible.

Action Plan

Include more fiber in your diet throughout the day but also at dinnertime. At dinner, you want to try and get your fiber from low carbohydrate foods. As you read earlier in this book, cutting down on carbohydrates at dinnertime is a great strategy for losing weight.

If you're coming up short on answers for foods that are high in fiber but also low in carbohydrates, here are some ideas for you:

- **Avocado**: an avocado is a nutrition goldmine. It's full of vitamins and minerals your body needs and it also happens to be delicious. Plus, it's got healthy, unsaturated fat, which you want to add in your dinner. Plus, one avocado has just 3 grams of carbohydrates but offers 12 grams of fiber. So, it is a great option for a low carbohydrate dinner.

- **Broccoli**: this is another great low carbohydrate option for dinner. One cup of chopped, cooked broccoli yields 16 grams of fiber with only 6 grams of carbohydrates. So, load up on broccoli for a nutritious, filling, low carbohydrate meal.

- **Cauliflower**: broccoli's tasty cousin is also a great low carbohydrate dinner option. One cup of these provides 4 grams of fiber with just 2 grams of carbohydrates. So, combine it with broccoli for a colorful, low carbohydrate plate.

- **Collard greens**: in one cup of cooked, chopped collard greens, you'll get 5 grams of fiber but only 4 grams of carbohydrates. You can stir these up into almost anything to add some nice texture and flavor to any meal.

In general, when you are looking for a low carbohydrate, high fiber food, you want to look for vegetables that aren't too starchy. Potatoes and corn are good examples of extremely starchy foods that you'll want to try and keep off your dinner plate. Although, you can welcome them onto your lunch plate! Aside from the low carbohydrate options above, beans, legumes, and whole grains are fantastic sources of fiber that also boast a high amount of protein as well. So, you can kill two birds with one nutritious stone if you add these to your meal. Actually, since they are also loaded with other vitamins and minerals, it's more like killing dozens of birds with one stone.

Everyday Habit #14

Curb Cravings with Nutrition (Part II)

In part II of our quest to fight cravings with nutrition, we will look at protein. Protein is a more complex nutrient than you might think. That's because it's not just one nutrient (like fiber or calcium). It's actually 9 separate amino acids that all work together. The reason you need to know that protein is built up of 9 essential amino acids is because not all protein sources contain the same amino acids. For example, if you tried to live entirely on beans as your protein source, you would become deficient in 2 of the essential amino acids that you need because beans don't provide you with all nine.

Fish, beef, chicken, and all other animal sources of protein do provide a complete spectrum of all 9 essential amino acids but if you ate exclusively beef as your source of protein, you'd get the high blood pressure and high cholesterol that come with it. So, it is important to eat a range of protein sources. For most plant sources of protein, you'll need to combine different sources to get all 9 essential amino acids. For example, if you eat beans, combine it with rice or corn. Rice and corn each have a higher amount of the 2 amino acids that beans are lacking while beans have a high supply of the amino acids that both rice and corn are lacking. You can also combine nuts and seeds with quinoa to create another delicious (and complete) protein.

Now, let's talk about how protein helps you lose weight. Usually when we think about fat burning diets, meat, beans, and nuts don't usually come to mind. These are rich, flavorful foods and diets usually demand that we get rid of flavor and suffer through our days surviving on plain lettuce. Eating only lettuce will make you lose weight but there's no reason to suffer when you can lose just as much weight while eating a delicious and healthy diet.

Protein is essential to that healthy, weight loss diet. This is because protein takes a long time for your body to break down and absorb. The longer it takes food to move through your digestive system, the longer you will feel full. Protein is, by far, the most difficult thing for your system to process so it spends the longest amount of time in your stomach. This will keep you feeling completely full all the way to your next meal. Because it also absorbs into your system more slowly, your blood glucose levels are stabilized so you don't experience a sudden crash. Sudden drops in the amount of glucose in your blood are a major cause of cravings. By avoiding the crash, you avoid the cravings that come with it.

Action Plan

You want to eat a lot of protein at dinner. By a lot, we are talking about 25 grams. This is the number one way to stave off late night cravings. Protein combined with low carbohydrate sources of fiber and unsaturated fats will keep your blood glucose levels as stabilized as possible while also keeping you feeling full. This means that your dinner will attack the two main causes of after dinner snacking. Good sources of protein include fish, poultry, chicken, beans, legumes, nuts, and seeds. Remember to combine your plant sources so that you get the full range of protein.

At dinner, your protein source (or sources if you're combining) should be the largest portion on your plate. The second largest should be your unsaturated fats. The smallest portion should be your fiber rich carbohydrates. If you're eating fish, you don't need to add any other fatty foods because fish are naturally rich in unsaturated fats. If you're eating beans or legumes, you don't need to add any other fiber sources because these are already high enough in fiber.

As you plan your meals for the week, make sure your dinner is the most protein rich meal of your day. Do this by eating a little less protein during breakfast and lunch so that you don't go overboard.

Remember, you need 50 grams of protein, 30 grams of fiber, and 20 grams of unsaturated fats. This is, of course, assuming you have no major health conditions that give you special dietary requirements. By making sure that you choose a variety of foods for each of these three things, you can make sure that you are also getting a good amount of the vitamins and minerals that you need.

In a single day, you should have at least 3 different sources of protein, 3 different sources of fiber, and 3 different sources of fat. Throughout the week, try to have 5 different sources of each one that you cycle through over the course of your week. This kind of variety not only helps you cover all your vitamins and minerals, it also keeps your diet from getting dull and boring. Variety is the spice of life, after all.

Everyday Habit #15

Establish Food-Free Zones

One good way to restrict when you eat is to restrict *where* you eat. When you eat in the living room or bedroom, it makes it easy to just grab a snack and mindlessly munch even when you're not hungry. We all do it and it seems like a harmless activity but it does actually cause some problems because you aren't paying attention to the signals your body is telling you. The more you ignore those "I've had enough" signals from your stomach, the more your body will start to ignore them, too. This makes it harder and harder to avoid overeating. By restricting the places in your house where food is allowed, you can make sure that you are always consciously deciding when you eat and how much you eat. You will become more aware of when you start to feel full and should stop. You'll also be able to actually enjoy the flavors more and avoid letting a whole bar of chocolate disappear without you even realizing you ate it all. Plus, it will mean no more crumbs on the bed or sofa!

Part of the logic behind this habit is that you have fewer opportunities to be distracted while eating. When you eat in the living room, it's usually because you are watching TV or surfing the Internet. On the other hand, if you had to get up from the couch and go to the kitchen every time you wanted to eat a handful of popcorn, you will be much less likely to snack. So, choosing one or two places in the house where food is allowed will make sure that you snack less and that you can make smarter choices about what you eat. You'll be paying more attention to the food and more attention to what your body is telling you, which will also help you recognize when you are full and avoid overeating. With that in mind, not just snacks but also all your meals during the day should be eaten in the same place.

Adopting this habit will reprogram your brain and body to know when it's time to eat. Once it becomes a habit, you will retrain your subconscious to associate that one place with eating. This will help regulate and moderate your appetite so that you only start to feel hungry when it's actually time to eat. You'll have fewer between meal cravings. This is the same logic behind evening habit #5 (make sleep a priority). Part of preparing for sleep is not doing other activities in the bed (like eating, watching TV, or working). This helps your subconscious realize that when it is in bed, it is time to go to sleep. The same thing is happening when you associate eating with only certain areas in the house.

Action Plan

The most logical place to eat is the kitchen or dining room. Your food-free zones should be absolutely everywhere else in the house. Don't bring food in the living room, bedroom, bathroom, laundry room, garage, or anywhere else. Prepare your meals in the kitchen and eat them sitting down at the table. While you are eating, don't watch TV or use the computer. Pay attention to your food. Eat slowly and savor the flavors. Make sure that you are sitting down while you eat. When you stand and eat, your body is in a constant state of feeling like it should be on the go. This makes it more difficult to eat slowly and focus only on eating. So, sit down, take your time, and let mealtime be a relaxing activity. Don't let it be a rushed or stressful part of your day. When you're done, clear the dishes and continue with your night. Doing anything else while you eat will lower your ability to recognize when you feel full. This means you'll have a tendency to overeat because you're just shoveling in food without giving your body the time it needs to send the signal to your brain that it's full. The second part of this habit is not using the kitchen or dining room for any other activity. If you have limited space in your home and you can't avoid using the dining table for other purposes as well, that's okay. Just make sure you don't do those other activities at the same time you are eating. If you can avoid it, though, it's best to make your kitchen and dining room "food-only" zones while the rest of your house becomes a "food-free" zone.

At work, avoid eating at your desk if you can. Use the break room or eat your lunch outside. Don't snack while you work. If you need to eat a snack, leave your desk to do it. Just like at home, your workspace should be a food-free zone. If your schedule allows for it, make sure you eat your meals in these places at the same time each day or at least within 30 minutes to an hour of a set time. The more structured your eating habits become, the less likely you will be to have sporadic cravings. Your stomach (well, technically, your subconscious) will learn that if it's not 7pm and you're not in the dining room, then it's not time to be hungry. This might be tough if you have kids who are used to snacking in front of the TV but remain firm. If you do, not only can you help yourself break this bad habit, you'll be helping your kids to build up these good, healthy habits now while they are still young. You'll thank yourself next time you're doing the dishes and you don't have to run all around the house looking for stray cups and plates. Not to mention you'll no longer have to deal with all the spills and stains on carpets, tables, and floors! Well, except in the kitchen or dining room, that is.

Everyday Habit #16

Know What Your Body Is Actually Telling You

The bad news is a craving for gummy bears doesn't mean your body is dangerously low on Vitamin Gummy. The good news is you can kill that gummy bear craving by eating a healthy alternative. You don't have to suffer through sweet tooth withdrawals if you know what your cravings actually mean. Eating a nutritious snack that provides the nutrients your body actually needs will get rid of that unhealthy craving and leave you feeling even more satisfied (and a whole lot less guilty!).

Cravings are not just random impulses to eat a certain food. They are actually signals your body is sending you to let you know what nutrients it's running low on at the moment. Unfortunately, the signal gets lost in translation very easily especially if you are used to a diet high in junk food. Your body can't tell you exactly what food it needs; all it can do is make you crave a certain range of flavors. That means it is up to you to decode the message and figure out what your cravings really mean. Each craving you have is a sign that you are low on a specific nutrient (or set of nutrients). By snacking on foods that contain those nutrients, you can get rid of the unhealthy craving that is making you suffer, give your body what it really needs, and keep your calories down in a healthy range all at the same time.

Action Plan

Put this knowledge to use by figuring out exactly which healthy foods will help fight which cravings and buying those healthy alternatives at the store instead of buying the unhealthy snacks you usually get. To help you correctly translate your cravings and find the healthy snack alternatives that will help you get rid of them, here is a quick chart that you can keep for easy reference:

What Your Craving:	What You Actually Need:	What You Should Eat:
Sugary Foods and Sweets	+ Chromium + Phosphorus + Tryptophan + Glucose (i.e.- you may have low blood sugar)	Nuts, seeds, beans, legumes, fresh fruit, eggs, dairy (High protein or natural sugars to stabilize glucose levels and restore nutrients)
Bready or Starchy Foods	+ Nitrogen	Nuts, beans, legumes, oatmeal, quinoa (High protein foods and high fiber foods)
Fatty Foods	+ Healthy, unsaturated fats + Calcium	Fish, nuts, seeds, legumes, beans, yogurt, avocado, broccoli, olive oil (Foods high in unsaturated fats or calcium)
Coffee or Caffeine	+ Phosphorus + Iron + Water (i.e.- you may be dehydrated*)	Nuts, legumes, eggs, poultry, beef, water (Drink water and eat high protein foods since they are also often high in

		phosphorus and iron)
Alcohol	+ Protein + Calcium + Potassium	Meat, nuts, seeds, legumes, beans, dark leafy greens, bananas, yogurt, squash, oatmeal (High protein foods and high mineral foods)
Carbonated Drinks	+ Calcium	Yogurt, legumes, broccoli, spinach, dark leafy greens, canned salmon (with bones), molasses (High calcium foods and also drink water)
Salty Foods	+ B vitamins + Vitamin C + Potassium + Decrease Stress**	Bananas, dark leafy greens, fish, liver, poultry, tomatoes, kiwis (Foods high in B vitamins, Vitamin C, or potassium)
Cigarettes	+ Silicon + Tyrosine	Nuts, seeds, legumes (Mineral rich, hearty foods. Also avoid refined flour, sugar, and starches)
Chocolate	+Magnesium	Dark chocolate (70%

65

| | +Glucose (low blood sugar again) | cocoa), fish, spinach, other dark leafy greens

(Foods with high magnesium content) |

*If you are craving a cup of coffee because you feel tired or groggy, you may actually be dehydrated. Studies show that drinking a glass or two of water when you hit that mid-afternoon lull could perk you up even more than a cup of coffee. Of course, if you're long time coffee drinker, you are probably also addicted to the caffeine but you should try to have a tall glass of water with your coffee.

**Salty food cravings are almost always a sign of excess stress hormones in the body, so you can also try stress reducing techniques like deep breathing, meditation, or calm walks in the park to reduce this craving. In addition to cravings, there are a few other symptoms of nutrition deficiency that your body is using to try and tell you to get more of a certain vitamin or mineral.

Here are three of the most common ones:

Symptom:	What You Actually Need:	What You Should Eat:
PMS	+ Zinc + Iron + Folate	Red meats (especially liver and other organ meats), seafood, dark leafy greens, carrots, turnips (High protein foods, especially meat and high fiber foods, especially root

		vegetables)
Loss of Appetite	+ B Vitamins + Manganese + Chloride	Red meat, nuts, seeds, beans, legumes, fish, blueberries, pineapple (High protein or mineral rich foods. If you also have nausea, try beef broths or fresh pineapple juice mixed with sparkling water)
Overeating, Binge Eating	+ Silicon + Tryptophan + Tyrosine	Nuts, seeds, liver, lamb, spinach, orange/green/red fruits and vegetables (High protein and mineral rich foods, high vitamin C. Also avoid refined flour, sugar, and starches)

The alternative snack options in this chart may not sound like they could possibly satisfy your cravings. I mean, who wants to eat fish when they're really craving donuts? But this chart is based on the science behind those cravings, not the flavors themselves. If you want donuts and you opt for a healthy sweet option like dried apricots, you're going to be disappointed. Not only are the apricots not as sugary and fluffy as a donut, they don't have the specific nutrient your body is actually craving.

So, while these foods might sound like they're in a whole different ballpark from your craving, eating them will actually stop the craving and make you feel more satisfied afterward. It will take some time to adapt to this healthy snacking habit, especially if you have formed an emotional or psychological dependency on the foods your craving. But if you stick with it and fight your cravings with healthy food, you will eventually reprogram your brain and correct the signal so that when your body is low on a certain nutrient, it can tell you to crave the right foods. Just watch, in a few weeks, you're going to find yourself actually craving broccoli!

Everyday Habit #17

Make After-Dinner Snacking Hard Work

When you feel like having a snack in the evening, it's very rarely because you are actually hungry. Most of that craving is just a simple habit. You are used to snacking so you keep snacking. This is especially the case when you are watching TV or doing some other activity while you eat.

It can be comforting or relaxing to just go through the motions of snacking. You might open a bag of cookies as you turn on the TV and before the first commercial break, it's empty and you hardly even remember eating that many cookies. It can be difficult to fight the urge to munch while you're watching your favorite show. This is one of the reasons that evening habit #12 is so important (watching less TV). Cutting down on the amount of TV you watch will help cut down on the amount of TV time snacking you do.

Of course, we all have our shows and no matter how much we want to lose weight, it's not worth giving up our favorite show! So, if you must find out what happens to your favorite characters and you can't resist the urge to snack while you watch, then pick snacks that are hard work. Slowing down the time between bites gives your body time to react and feel full (as you read in the first chapter). It also lets you indulge in the act of snacking without consuming as many calories since you're not shoveling in bite after bite. Instead, you're eating at a slow, even pace, with plenty of breaks in between.

Action Plan

Instead of cookies, go for pistachios in the shell. The time it takes you to break the shell open will help slow down your eating and cut down on the total amount of calories you consume while watching TV. Some other good hard-work snacking options include oranges, pomegranates, cherries with the pit in, sunflower seeds in the shell, oranges with the peel on. You can also get a nutcracker and go for walnuts, pecans, and other shelled nuts. Bringing tools into your snack time will take it to a whole new level! Another way to make snacking hard work is to take a food that is simple to eat and make it more difficult. Instead of biting into a whole apple, take a knife with you and cut slices out one at a time. Keep a glass of water with you and take a drink from it between every bite. Whichever method you choose, make sure your snacks are still healthy. Eating cookies slowly might mean fewer cookies, but they're still cookies. Try to choose

Everyday Habit #18

"Serving Size" Is Not Just a Suggestion

This habit sounds simple but it can actually be pretty challenging. You know that serving size mentioned on the package of your favorite snack? For a box of cookies, the serving size is probably something like 1 or 2 cookies. Well, when you want to eat a sugary, junky snack, eat only a single serving. Don't take the whole box of cookies with you, just pull out a single serving. This will help you cut down on junk food and sweets (and slowly start eliminating them or only eating them on special occasions) without having to totally give it all up at once.

Action Plan

If you have had a craving for chips that's lasted hours and you just don't have the willpower to fight it anymore, go ahead and have some chips. But first check the packaging to see how many chips are in a single serving. Remove that amount of chips from the bag and put the rest of the bag away. Eat your chips slowly...savor them.

Everyday Habit #19

Start Snack-Free Shopping

The grocery store is where your battle to cut calories begins. Studies have proven that people are more likely to have cravings for foods that are close to them and readily available. If you know you've got a secret stash of cookies hiding in the kitchen, it's going to take all of your mental energy to resist devouring them. But if there aren't any cookies to eat, you'll be less likely to have cravings for them. Of course, you will start to miss them but the craving won't be as strong as if they were in your house, whispering your name, beckoning you to come enjoy just one little bite.

Ban snacks (especially junk food) from your grocery cart and avoid having to face your greatest temptations every night when you get home. The food that you have in your house should only be ingredients for meals. If it's ready to eat, don't buy it. The exception to that rule is, of course, fruits and vegetables that you can eat raw. Don't buy chips, cookies, soda, crackers, candy, granola bars, or anything like that. You should even avoid the "healthy" snacks because the goal here is to break your snacking habit.

There are some foods that are ready to eat and totally snack-worthy that you might consider if you've got a serious habit and don't feel like you're ready to give up snacking all at once. Here is a quick list of foods that burn more calories than they actually contain (because chewing and digesting use up more calories than the amount in the food):

1. **Celery**: if you skip the peanut butter and eat them plain, celery is 75% water and 25% water. Because of this, 1 large stalk (about 12 inches long) contains just 10 calories. You'll burn that just from chewing. Even more calories will be burned as you digest it. Plus, the high amount of fiber will help you digest and help you feel fuller. It's also full of vitamins. So you can snack totally guilt free.

2. **Grapefruit**: these vitamin-rich gems contain 51 calories, which may sound like you can't burn it all from eating, but grapefruit actually boosts your metabolism! Plus, you have to peel it, pull it apart, chew it, and digest it so all the calories burned does add up. The high fiber content will also leave you feeling satisfied while you boost your immune system and lower your cholesterol!

3. **Watermelon**: this fruit is delicious so it probably won't take much convincing to get you to add it to your cart. But you'll be pleased to learn that because watermelon is (not surprisingly) mostly water, it contains very few calories. It's also got (more surprisingly) protein. Between the protein and fiber, you'll be able to feel full without adding any calories since digestion burns more than the amount watermelon has to start with.

4. **Broth**: vegetable broth, beef broth, any kind of broth will give you that nice warm, savory flavor you look for in a hearty meal without all the calories that usually come with it. So if you must snack after dinner and it must be something substantial, opt for a bowl of warm broth instead. The warmth will be soothing, the flavor will satisfy your tongue, and you'll even get some nutrition from it as well!

5. **Apples**: biting, chewing, and digesting an apple all require more calories than you'll actually find in the apple itself. They're a sweet, high fiber treat that will fill you up without fattening you up. Plus, one study showed that eating apples daily could reduce your risk by as much as 17%! It turns out an apple a day really does keep the doctor away.

6. **Chili Peppers**: while you probably don't feel like munching down on a chili pepper by itself, slicing them up and adding them to another snack (or to your main meals) is a great way to boost your metabolism. Capsaicin (the compound in peppers that gives them their kick) is scientifically proven to increase metabolism and help you burn more calories. Slice them up and mix them into a bowl of vegetables or fruits (sugar and spice are made for each other!). Make a spicy salsa and dollop it on some lettuce for a low calorie, metabolism boosting treat!

7. **Tomatoes**: these are a delicious low-calorie option that packs a lot of flavor and a lot of vitamins. Plus, it's the perfect base to that salsa you're going to make!

Action Plan

Make a shopping list before you go to the store. The list should be snack-free, of course! The best way to make a shopping list is to first plan out all of your meals for the week (or the month, depending on how often you go to the store).

Figure out exactly what ingredients you need and how much of each ingredient you need. Then, when you get to the store, buy only those ingredients and only enough for your meals. You can actually save a lot of money this way and not just from cutting out snacks. If you plan meals that share ingredients, you can buy some things in bulk and save money.

Plan nutritious meals that are high in fiber and protein so that they keep you feeling full and satisfied even between meals. Don't stress too much about the calorie counts on your main meals. The most important thing is the nutrition value. If you're getting enough nutrition from your main meals, you'll be less likely to snack in between. So, don't buy low-fat or low-calorie versions of your ingredients. Moderate amounts of unsaturated fats are an important part of a balanced diet and can also help you feel more satisfied after your meal. Since you'll be cutting out between meal snacks, you can afford to add a few extra calories to your main meals in the name of satisfaction, nutrition and flavor!

To sum it all up, this should be your new grocery shopping routine:

1. Plan all of your meals for the week (breakfast, lunch, and dinner).

    a. Make sure they are high fiber, high protein meals made from unprocessed foods

2. Write out a list of all the ingredients

    a. Include the exact amount of each ingredient that you need to make all of your meals

3. Go to the store and buy exactly what is on your list.

    a. No extras and no splurges. Walk right past that snack isle and don't look back!

If you are still not confident that a nutritious meal is enough to get you through the day without snacking, buy some of the options suggested above so that you can snack without adding calories.

Everyday Habit #20

Track Your Progress and Stay Motivated

Tracking your progress is more about making sure you stay on course and don't lose sight of your goals but this is an important part of losing weight. If you don't keep track of how well you've been doing, you'll be less likely to stick with your weight loss habits in the long run. Keeping track can also help make sure you don't forget anything. When you are juggling a lot of new habits at once (even if you are doing it one step at a time), it can be difficult to remember all the new things you are doing.

Get a notebook or keep a file on your computer for keeping a daily record of your progress. You can look through it at the end of each week to see how well you've done, figure out where you might need to make some improvements, and just generally take pride in the fact that you are committing to making this change in your life. This can be a major source of motivation because in the daily struggle of trying to adopt healthier habits, every little setback might feel like an insurmountable obstacle. But when you take the time to look back and see that you have actually managed to do surprisingly well (even with a few slip ups here and there), you'll have the encouragement you need to keep going for the next week.

As the weeks add up and you see that you've got over a month of progress recorded, you'll be able to see how far you have actually come. Habits that seemed completely impossible to keep up with at the beginning could become some of your favorite routines. Journaling throughout this experience of making healthy changes to your lifestyle is also a great activity to do in the evening. Not only is it a stimulating activity that will keep you distracted from snacking, it's also a great way to stay motivated even at night (which is when our energy and willpower are usually at their lowest).

Action Plan

Your progress journal can include whatever information you feel is the most important to keep track of but here are some ideas of the sort of things you could include:

- Number of calories you've eaten
- Number of calories burned
- Number of calories you *haven't* eaten
- Amount of weight lost (do this weekly rather than daily)
- Amount of money spent on food
- Amount of money *saved* on food
- Brief descriptions of your mood, energy levels, changes in your physical or emotional wellbeing, or just how you are feeling about the challenge you have chosen to take on

Create a journal entry template with space for each of the things you want to include and fill it out every evening. You can do it as soon as you get home from your post-meal evening walk! At the end of every week, as you record your new weight, take some time to look back through the records for each day. You can do a weekly tally of how many calories you didn't eat and write down a few notes about what your goals are for the week ahead. Create a template for reflecting so that you can make a conscious effort to thoroughly reflect on your progress each week. Include questions like these:

1. What was my biggest accomplishment last week?
2. What was my greatest challenge last week?
3. Did I meet all of my goals for the week?
4. What do I want to accomplish next week?
5. What might be my greatest challenges next week?
6. What are some strategies I can use to overcome those challenges?

A thorough system for keeping track of your progress will help you stay on track and be a constant source of motivation. The achievements you have made might not be easy to notice as they happen gradually from day to day but when you have them written down on paper, you will be surprised how far you have come in such a short amount of time.

Everyday Habit #21

Take the 30-Day Weight Loss Challenge

This last habit is not so much a daily habit as a way for you to adopt the other 20 habits you have read about in this book. By slowly adding in these healthy habits, you can help make sure that you don't lose focus or motivation. Some of these are big changes and when you combine them all, that's a dramatic change to your current lifestyle. If you attempted to do it all at once, you'd find it impossible to juggle them all and lose hope pretty quickly. You can create your own 30-day challenge that works better for you but the plan suggested here is an effective way to help you adopt each habit and make sure that it sticks.

Tweak the plan as needed to suit your own situation but don't overburden yourself. Also, don't make it too easy on yourself. This is going to be a challenge no matter how you tackle it. So, find a good, steady pace that works for you. This 30-day weight loss challenge is not meant to help you lose all the weight in 30 days and then go back to your old lifestyle. These are habits you should keep for a lifetime so that the weight comes off and stays off for good. If you stick to it, you will notice dramatic results after your first 30 days. You are going to lose a lot of water weight and burn a high amount of fat.

As you start to get muscle, the weight will begin to drop more slowly. This is not because your fat is deciding to stick around but because muscle just weighs more than fat. Even if your scale begins to slow down, your waistline is going to continue to shrink. So as you are tracking your progress, remember to measure your waist as well as recording your weight so you can keep a more accurate measure of your progress.

Day 1	Habit #1
Day 2	Habit #1
Day 3	Habit #1
Day 4	Habit #1 Habit #2
Day 5	Habit #1 Habit #2
Day 6	Habit #1 Habit #2
Day 7	Habit #1 Habit #2 Habit #3
Day 8	Habit #1 Habit #2 Habit #3
Day 9	Habit #1 Habit #2 Habit #3
Day 10	Habit #1 Habit #2 Habit #3 Habit #4
Day 11	Habit #1 Habit #2 Habit #3 Habit #4
Day 12	Habit #1 Habit #2 Habit #3 Habit #4
Day 13	Habit #1 Habit #2 Habit #3 Habit #4 Habit #5
Day 14	Habit #1 Habit #2 Habit #3 Habit #4 Habit #5
Day 15	Habit #1 Habit #2 Habit #3 Habit #4 Habit #5
Day 16	Habit #1 Habit #2 Habit #3 Habit #4 Habit #5 Habit #6
Day 17	Habit #1 Habit #2 Habit #3 Habit #4 Habit #5 Habit #6
Day 18	Habit #1 Habit #2 Habit #3 Habit #4 Habit #5 Habit #6
Day 19	Habit #1 Habit #2 Habit #3 Habit #4 Habit #5 Habit #6 Habit #7
Day 20	Habit #1 Habit #2 Habit #3 Habit #4 Habit #5 Habit #6 Habit #7
Day 21	Habit #1 Habit #2 Habit #3 Habit #4 Habit #5 Habit #6 Habit #7
Day 22	Habit #1 Habit #2 Habit #3 Habit #4 Habit #5 Habit #6 Habit #7 Habit #8
Day 23	Habit #1 Habit #2 Habit #3 Habit #4 Habit #5 Habit #6 Habit #7 Habit #8
Day 24	Habit #1 Habit #2 Habit #3 Habit #4 Habit #5 Habit #6

	Habit #7 Habit #8
Day 25	Habit #1 Habit #2 Habit #3 Habit #4 Habit #5 Habit #6 Habit #7 Habit #8 Habit #9
Day 26	Habit #1 Habit #2 Habit #3 Habit #4 Habit #5 Habit #6 Habit #7 Habit #8 Habit #9
Day 27	Habit #1 Habit #2 Habit #3 Habit #4 Habit #5 Habit #6 Habit #7 Habit #8 Habit #9
Day 28	Habit #1 Habit #2 Habit #3 Habit #4 Habit #5 Habit #6 Habit #7 Habit #8 Habit #9 Habit #10
Day 29	Habit #1 Habit #2 Habit #3 Habit #4 Habit #5 Habit #6 Habit #7 Habit #8 Habit #9 Habit #10
Day 30	Habit #1 Habit #2 Habit #3 Habit #4 Habit #5 Habit #6 Habit #7 Habit #8 Habit #9 Habit #10

Continue adding one habit every fourth day for the next 30 days as well and you will have all 20 healthy evening habits established. By the third month, they will become so engrained that you will hardly have to think about doing them. They will just come naturally and be part of your new lifestyle that will help you lose weight and be healthier overall.

Bonus Tips

Weight loss is a topic that many people have trouble approaching and so is healthy eating. This is not because they don't want to lose weight and eat healthy, but because of how much effort it takes and because they feel like they have to make sudden, dramatic changes in their life. It is easy to become comfortable in the way you are living. Especially if you have been eating unhealthy and living a life that is drained from energy for a long period of time. You no longer remember what you are missing and this has become your safe zone.

Eating is also a deeply personal activity, even if you eat with your family or at a restaurant. For many people, it is just as personal as their relationship with other people. People who have this mental approach to food also find it difficult to talk about their eating habits, as it is part of their private life.

Making a Change

Making a change in your life can be difficult. This means that you have to carefully analyze your current lifestyle and be honest with yourself and your support system about your current habits and the ones that you plan to change. The larger your support system is, the more successful you will be in achieving your goals. Getting the people that you live with – your family, your children, and your spouse to follow the concept of a healthy lifestyle can dramatically increase your chances of success. It can be difficult to get children to follow a healthier lifestyle, but it can be achieved with persistence and educating them about the food that they are eating, as well as allowing them to help you cook or prepare the food.

Dramatic Changes Are Not Necessary

The truth is, you don't have to make dramatic changes, or a lot of changes all at once to live a better life. By simply changing one habit at a time, you can make a world of difference in your current weight, and begin melting the fat away without causing any stress in your life. As you feel better about yourself, these changes directly affect your life in a positive way and you will see that small changes in your daily habits can make a huge impact on your life. Losing weight is not always about completing a grueling workout on a daily basis. Sometimes, it is simply changing your personal habits, one by one, step by step.

What bad habits do you have that contribute to your current weight? Many people are not aware of how many habits they have that pack on the pounds, and because of this, they fight a losing battle with the treadmill, eventually giving up on losing weight altogether. The tips that are shared in this book are meant to be instated one at a time to ensure your success. Try each daily habit change for at least one to two weeks before introducing a new habit to your daily regimen.

Building and Breaking Habits

According to research, it takes close to 14 days to make or break a habit. Because of this, you will only want to start one new habit at a time. Make sure that you have created a habit fully before proceeding to the next. This is the best way to ensure your success through your weight loss journey. The key to losing weight and keeping it off is to lose weight in a slow and effective manner. Losing weight too fast or making too many changes in your daily routine can cause you to give up, or lose track of your true goals, as well as put unnecessary strain on your everyday life.

Make Sure Your Weight Loss Efforts Are Stress Free

By making changes in your life slowly, you are ensuring your personal success. This is because you create less stress in your life. Excess stress can cause weight gain and counteract the positive effects of your hard work and dedication. This is because the hormones that are released when you are stressed directly contribute to weight gain, and can do so in a very short period of time. Before you begin instating new habits, try to remove as much stress as possible from your life. Create a schedule and stick to it. Read through this book completely and determine which changes will make the most impact in your life and map out your personal goals in a way that your lifestyle supports.

Enjoy the Benefits

The best part of making a change in your life, is taking time to enjoy the benefits. If you need motivation to get started, pick one of the tips in this book that means the most to you. Utilize this tip over a period of one month. See what benefits you get from following the advice that follows it. Then, you will see how easy it is to lose weight by changing a few things in your current life, instead of changing your *entire* life.

Living Healthier

Eating healthy foods gives you longer lasting boost of energy. It also helps you to feel better about yourself as you develop healthier looking skin and hair. Feeling great translates to the way you approach life, work and fun creating a better balance in your life. As you feel better physically and mentally, your confidence will shine through and you will notice a drastic increase in the amount of effort you are willing to put into developing new, healthy habits on a regular basis.

A Healthier You Makes for a Happier You

The healthier you are, the better you feel about life in general. You are more likely to stay in shape, eat right, and take advantage of developing a well-rounded social life.

When you feel healthy, it shows through every action you take. You will be able to adapt healthy habits easier and over time, you will notice that your life has taken on a more positive vibe. Before you know it, you will notice a positive change in all aspects of your life, including your relationships and your finances.

Increased Energy

Eating healthy and staying active allows you to develop more energy and maintain your energy level longer. You will notice that you have more stamina and endurance to get through your daily routine with plenty of positive energy left for a great evening with friends or family.

Enjoying Life!

Our purpose in producing this book was to share ways that you can lose weight, have more energy, live a healthy life and enjoy life to its fullest. Life is not worth living if you cannot enjoy time with family, friends, and your own routine. Also, actually enjoying life can translate into feeling positive about new experiences and creating new habits. You can begin enjoying life again by taking small, simple steps toward developing healthy habits that last for a lifetime. We know you will love the way you feel as you begin to change your habits.

Most people do not realize how much their habits drain their energy and their life of positive feelings and positive changes. You will notice at each change that your life becomes easier, smoother and overall better. This is your own confidence at work and your body thanking you for finally taking the steps you need to live a healthy, happy, energy filled, successful life.

Learning New Habits

Learning new habits can take between 14 to 21 days. This is why it is essential for you to pay attention to your subconscious habits and whether you are carrying out these actions without thinking. If you have accomplished the ability to carry out the action without thinking about it, or talking yourself into it, you have developed a new, positive habit.

Children and Obesity

While many experts point their finger at the United States for leading children into obesity, there are obese children all over the world; just as there are starving children scattered throughout the world. Rather than blaming the world or certain countries, we have to take accountability for our own lives and the future of our own children. By starting positive habits in our own lives, while our children are young enough to observe our habits and take them in on their own, we impress upon them that a certain way of life is ideal. Eating right, staying active, taking vitamins and visiting your doctor regularly become instilled in their personality. While this is ideal, it is not always easy to make these changes while your children are young enough to grow up knowing only healthy foods and a certain way of life.

Sometimes, it takes reprograming your entire family to live a better life and while most children are not on board for giving up that bag of potato chips, it is your job as a parent to make these foods inaccessible while your children are learning a new way of life, and introducing them to a way of life that will make them feel better, and leave a long-lasting result.

Teaching Children New Habits

Teaching children new habits may seem difficult at first. However, you should ensure that if your children are old enough, you should take the time to explain to them why you have made the decision, and let them know that it is important to give the changes a chance and then allow them to determine how they feel after the changes are made.

It is also important to note that even resistant children will evolve over time and the habits will be made subconsciously after a short duration of time. This is for many reasons:

1. They are hungry and the food they are being offered may be healthy, but it will fill their belly.

2. They must eat and if the only food they are offered is nutritious, they will choose food over being hungry.

While you may feel that your child initially rejecting the diet change is hopeless or cruel, you must also understand that your child's pediatrician would support your change to a healthier lifestyle, and that making your child eat healthy foods is not abusive, neglectful, or bad parenting – unless you are forcing them to eat something they are allergic to!

Remember That Depravation is Not Necessary

Through your efforts to lose weight, feel better, and omit foods that are less than desirable in your diet. You should make sure that you do not deprive yourself of the simple joys in life. We are not saying to eat pie daily, but a slice of pie every now and then will not completely destroy your diet. The key is to learn to enjoy these foods in moderation without over indulging. You are retraining your body to see these foods as treats instead of simply daily necessities as you currently do. You are teaching your body that healthy food comes first, and treats come later, just as your mother always told you!

Your Adjustment Period

As you know, with any diet change, you should expect your body to react differently to the foods that you are taking in. It is important that you expect the changes that your body will go through. Your digestive system may experience some upset, and you may find yourself needing to use the restroom more often than you previously did. You may also find yourself hungry more often, which can easily be remedied with negative calorie foods throughout the day to make up for the ease of digestion of the new foods you will be eating on a regular basis.

Everyday Habit #22

Focus on Vegetables

One of the number one reasons people have trouble eating right is because determining serving sizes can be difficult. Who really has time for the entire math that goes into weighing, adding, estimating, and measuring their food? How many pieces of lettuce fit in a cup? How many pieces of broccoli equal a serving size? The truth is that life is busy and nobody really has time for that much detail. No matter how good you get at measuring your food, you will never remember all of the measurements and this can stand in the way of you really enjoying life and enjoying your food.

Eating dinner with your family should be enjoyable and should not be a chore. Not to mention nothing makes you feel like you are on a diet more than pulling out a measuring cup to serve dinner. Feeling like you are on a diet can be oppressive, even more than the diet is and measuring makes the restrictions even worse. The great news is - you don't have to measure!

There is an easier way to determine your portion sizes, and it does not involve weighing, measuring or driving yourself insane. Simply fill half of your plate with vegetables and then divide the other half into two sections to accommodate your serving of protein and carbohydrates. Determining serving sizes becomes so much easier, and so does enjoying life.

You can eat out with friends, attend dinner parties, or host a dinner party without feeling like you have to measure or weigh your food, or that you are the strange obsessive person that carries around measuring cups in their purse to prepare their plate. Not only does this method give you the correct serving sizes, it also allows you to enjoy more freedom and less restriction while eating.

Do Not Center in on Single Vegetables

Focusing on single vegetables can cause your food to be bland and can cause your diet to lack essential nutrients that can be found in a variety of vegetables. Ensure that each plate you make has a wide variety of fresh vegetables that have been cooked to an al'dente state. Over cooking your vegetables, or cooking them until they no longer have resistance diminishes the nutritional value of the vegetables and can deplete them of essential minerals that your body needs.

Best Methods of Cooking Vegetables

The best method of cooking your vegetables is to sauté or steam them. Vegetables should never be microwaved or overcooked. Microwaving and overcooking vegetables removes most of the vitamin content from them and can dramatically reduce the benefit that you experience from them as well as alter the flavor.

ACTION PLAN

This simple method of setting up your plate is easy to do and feels less restrictive than weighing and measuring your food. The less you feel as though you are on a diet, the more successful you will be in developing new, healthier eating habits that you can stick with on a regular basis. Simply remember to fill half your plate with vegetables and split the other half of your plate with protein and a whole grain carbohydrate and you will be on your way to a healthier, thinner you in no time.

*Note: While they are available, the steam in bag, microwavable vegetables lose their nutritional value as they cook. Avoid these if possible. Always use a true vegetable steamer, or a pot of boiling water with a colander to steam them. If you feel your vegetables need more flavors, there are a variety of spices that you can use on them, including sea salt.

Everyday Habit #23
Increase This & See Results Immediately!

Not only can fiber help keep your digestive tract functioning correctly and keep your heart healthy, it is also a great way to help you lose weight. So, what is fiber? Fiber is a naturally occurring mineral in food that helps you feel full. Fiber also allows you to stay full for a longer period of time compared to other fillers, which helps you to avoid unhealthy food options that contain chemically created fillers when you are in a pinch.

Making sure that you get the correct amount of fiber everyday can ensure that you do not develop digestive backup, that the nutrients your body needs are completely removed from your food, and that you stools remain soft and easier to pass.

Fact about Constipation

Constipation is one of the leading causes of weight gain that most people face. It is also the number one cause of colon cancer among middle-aged men and women. Buildup of waste in your body can contribute to you feeling sluggish, drained and overall, unbalanced. It can also cause your body to randomly deposit fats in your problem areas.

Eating enough fiber everyday can prevent constipation and waste build up in your body. It can also help provide you with the energy necessary to get up, get moving and feel better about your overall health and the future of your health.

ACTION PLAN

To ensure that you are getting enough fiber in your diet, you should ensure that you are eating sources that are known for providing healthy fiber.

Fruits, vegetables and whole grain carbohydrates are packed with healthy fiber that will fuel your body and help you to develop better health in a very short period of time.

Make sure that you add up how much fiber you have taken in every day. Ensure that you ingest between 25 to 30 grams of fiber daily to ensure that you are creating a healthy digestive process. Don't have time for counting fiber intake? Fiber supplements are available over the counter and can be taken in capsule, tablet, and mixed-drink form.

Everyday Habit #24

Add Healthy Oil to Every Meal

No two oils are created equally. It isn't just that they are not created equally; a single type of oil cannot be used for all purposes. This is due to the chemical makeup, the flavor and the amount of heat it can withstand before scorching. Because of this, you should keep a wide variety of oils on hand and plan your meals according to their uses.

By adding two teaspoons of healthy oils to your meals, you increase the effectiveness of your digestion and make it easier for your body to derive the nutrients it needs from your food. At the same time, it gets rid of what you don't need to have stored in your body. We have created a delicious cheat sheet for you to use alongside your menu.

Healthy Baking Oils

The best healthy oils to bake with are coconut oil, palm oil, canola oil and high oleic safflower or sunflower oil.

Healthy Frying Oils

High quality, healthy oils for frying are avocado oil, peanut oil, palm oil, and sesame oil. They hold up great to the heat that is required when you fry foods and they are delicious.

Healthy Oils for Sautéing

Oils that are great for sautéing are avocado oil, canola oil, coconut oil, grape seed oil, olive oil, sesame oil and high oleic safflower and sunflower oils.

Healthy Oils for Dipping and Making Dressings and Marinades

When you are looking for a healthy dipping, dressing, or marinade oil, flavor cannot be compromised, but your health can not be compromised either. This is why we recommend flax oil, olive oil, peanut oil, toasted sesame seed oil, or walnut oil.

ACTION PLAN

Keeping healthy oils on hand is a great idea. However, you must also think of shelf life. Oils do diminish in quality and flavor over time, so only keep what you need at the time on hand. Make sure to plan your oils accordingly and purchase in small quantities at a time. This ensures that the oil is fresh and tastes great when you use it.

When you are creating your meal plan and grocery list, consider how you plan to cook each meal. This will help you to determine exactly what oils and how much of each you should have on hand to prepare your meals. Pay attention to the shelf life of the oil and refrigerate it if you plan to wait a significant amount of time before using it. While not all oils have to be refrigerated, it can help increase their shelf life and preserve their flavor.

Everyday Habit #25

Balance Your Protein and Carbs

The majority of your diet should consist of proteins and whole grain carbohydrates. You should ensure that every meal you eat has a serving of both, along with at least two tablespoons of a healthy fat source.

Proteins

Each serving of protein should be equivalent to the size of a deck of playing cards. Instead of focusing on weighing your protein source, learn to recognize a healthy serving of protein by looking at it. This will make eating out, eating at dinner parties and eating at friends' houses more comfortable and relaxed. Look at your protein source from all angles. It should be as tall, as wide and as deep as a deck of playing cards.

Carbohydrates

The serving size in relation to carbohydrates is a little more difficult to determine. Before deciding your serving size, you must first determine what category your carbohydrates fall into.

Grains: The average serving size for grain-based carbohydrates is approximately one ounce. For example: one slice of whole grain bread, one cup of prepared breakfast cereal, or ½ cup of cooked rice is considered a serving. You should consume between five to eight servings of grain-based carbohydrates per day.

Legumes: Legumes are considered both a protein and a carbohydrate. The main carbohydrate that they add to your diet is dietary fiber. One half cup of beans or peas is equivalent to one serving of vegetables, or two ounces of protein. Your weekly intake of bean-based intake should be between one to two cups.

Vegetables and Fruits: Vegetables and fruits are a great source of healthy carbohydrates. ½ cup of vegetables, or a full cup of raw leafy greens is considered a serving. You should have at least two to three cups of vegetable-based carbohydrates in your daily diet. A serving of fruit is considered a single piece of fruit. You should make sure to add at least 1-½ cups of fruit to your diet each day.

ACTION PLAN

While this is a lot to take in at first, you can easily adjust your diet a little at a time. Do not rush into changing your diet all at once. Take one step at a time and plan your meals and snacks wisely. There are many different websites that are geared toward helping people develop new, healthy menu habits. These resources can save a lot of time in planning your meals, and creating your grocery lists to accommodate your new diet.

If you feel overwhelmed at any point in your diet change, slow down and relax. It is not a race and the only winner is you! There are a lot of support groups that can help you get through rough patches in your diet change, even if you are trying to navigate a lifestyle change with children involved. There are thousands of people all over the world who will understand your struggles, lend advice that has worked for them, and even help you to come up with custom solutions that work for you. While you are making changes to your life, a support group can do wonders in helping you to stick with your plan, even if it is an online support group.

I hope that you are enjoying this book so far, and if you could spare 30 seconds, I would greatly appreciate you leaving a review on Amazon.com.

Everyday Habit #26

Take a Fish Oil Supplement

Fish oil is an amazing supplement for those who want to lose weight. This is because fish oil is a great source of Omega 3, an essential fatty acid that your body cannot create; it must be taken in through foods and supplements. Omega 3 fatty acids are a great way to flush impurities from the body, as well as assist in fat burning efforts that you already have in place.

Omega 3's not only help burn fat, but they also help reduce the amount of fat that your body is able to store over time, which increases your resistance to additional fat build up. You are probably wondering, if fish oil contains fat, how does it help me burn fat? Simply put, there is a huge difference in the way your body responds to saturated and unsaturated fats.

Unsaturated fats work with your body to increase your health and keep you healthy. Saturated fats bring you down, cause unhealthy effects, and cause you to gain weight. Taking in healthy fats on a regular basis can help you to regulate your blood sugar, even if you are not diabetic. The more stable your blood sugar is, the easier it is for your body to break down sugars and fats that are typically stored in the body.

Fish Oil and Your Exercise Plan

While fish oil is great for burning fat, many people overlook the advantage that a supplement provides when they are working out. The more muscle mass you have, the easier it is to burn fat during your workout. Fish oil helps to speed up metabolism, supports a healthy nutrient sorting process in the digestive system, and helps to build new muscle as you work out. This means that it helps you burn fat in multiple ways every day. Because of the number of ways fish oil helps just in weight loss, it is definitely worth taking two gel caps every day.

Fish Oil and Your Heart

As we talked about earlier in our tips, the more effective your blood flow is, the easier it is for your body to get rid of fat. Fish oil helps to increase your cardiovascular health and improves blood flow. This makes transporting the fat you burn to an exit point easier, more effective and more efficient. There are many other benefits to a fish oil supplement, but these are the ways it can help you lose weight and keep it off.

Omega 3 as a Vegetarian

DHA is a vitamin that is extremely high in the vegetarian diet. While you may not be getting Omega 3 directly from your food, your body has the ability to turn part of the DHA you take in into a product that is similar to Omega 3 fatty acid and your body will be able to use it as such.

However, in order to reach the daily requirements, you must take in a substantial amount of DHA each day in order for your body to create enough Omega 3 fatty acid to sustain your muscles.

ACTION PLAN

Just like with any supplement, it is important to find one that provides a quality fish oil. This is not a cheap adventure and a quality supplement is going to cost a lot more than the discount fish oil supplements that you are used to seeing. Some research may be necessary in order to find a supplement that suits your budget and high-quality standards. A quality fish oil supplement should be:

1. All Natural
2. Easy to Take
3. Made with Certified Ingredients
4. Created by a trusted manufacturer

Make sure not to purchase a supplement that is plant based. True Omega 3 oils can only be found in meat-based sources and can be found in their strongest and purest state in lean fat fish, like Salmon and halibut. If you are a vegetarian, you may want to take a DHA supplement in order to reach your maximum daily value to ensure that your muscles are strong, resilient and are able to absorb other nutrients.

Everyday Habit #27

The FUN Habit with MANY Benefits

While getting a massage once a month seems like pampering yourself instead of a weight loss effort and life changing effort, it can greatly reduce your stress. Stress creates hormones that allow your body to store fat easier. Getting a massage at least once per month can greatly reduce the amount of stress that you experience on a regular basis and increase your mood and activity level. This is a great way to lose weight and relax at the same time.

The more relaxed you are and the less you experience chronic stress, the easier it is to lose weight, even over a short period of time. Studies have shown a direct correlation between the levels of stress you feel, the way you manage it, and the amount of weight you retain and gain. When you combine this habit with others that we have listed in this book, you will notice dramatic changes in the way you feel and the way that you respond to stressful situations.

Getting a Massage from Your Partner Verses a Professional

While getting a massage from your partner is a welcome addition to any lifestyle, it is recommended that at least one massage per month come from a professional masseuse or massage therapist.

Make sure that your masseuse is aware that you are there to help reduce your stress level in an effort to lose weight. Certain massage methods are more effective in for this purpose than others and they will know what type of massage to recommend.

Overall Stress Reduction

While massage is a great way to reduce your stress, you should take advantage of other methods of stress reduction that will help you to avoid weight gain. Methods like following a schedule, limiting your daily duties, delegating duties when possible, and ensuring that you have enough time to eat relaxing meals and get plenty of sleep.

Make sure that you do not overbook yourself, and make sure that you meditate on a regular basis. With careful organization, planning and scheduling, you can dramatically reduce your stress beyond what a massage can offer. The massage acts as a bonus to these efforts, and can be looked at as a reward and a bonus stress relief.

ACTION PLAN

Make sure to schedule your massage for around the same time each month to ensure the best results and continuous results. If you notice that you need a massage more often in the beginning, pamper yourself twice per month until you start to see results.

Do not forget to create a schedule that you can stick to and fulfill on a daily basis. The more you are able to reduce your stress, the better your weight loss results will be. If you need help creating a schedule that will work for you, confer with your friends to create a support system and help you to devise a schedule that will work for you, your family, and the rest of your life.

Everyday Habit #28

Eat Dessert

What? What do I mean, "eat dessert?" Aren't I meant to be telling you to eat healthier? The truth is, by denying yourself dessert, you can make yourself feel deprived. One of the top reasons that people fail at losing weight is by giving up; and one of main reasons they give up is because they deprive themselves of the simple joys in life. By adhering to portion size, and enjoying a small dessert, you feel as though you are still able to enjoy life and enjoy that social time after a meal that dessert brings.

How to Allow Dessert

Allowing dessert to fit into your daily calorie count is simple. By allotting negative calorie foods as snack foods throughout the day, and focusing on healthy fat sources, you can easily reserve the calories that are contained in a dessert serving.

Stick to Dark Chocolates

Sticking to dark chocolates, rather than semi-sweet chocolate desserts, will reduce the calories contained in your dessert and allow you to enjoy a larger serving size. Dark chocolates provide a mild sweetness, but are not overbearing.

Dark chocolates contain approximately 20% sugar content while semi-sweet chocolate is comprised of approximately 35% sugar by volume. As you can see, this simple change can dramatically reduce the amount of calories that you consume in the average dessert.

Chocolate Cheat Sheet	
Type of Chocolate	**Sugar Concentration by Volume**
Dark Chocolate	20% Sugar by Volume
Semi-sweet chocolate	50% Sugar by Volume
Bitter-sweet chocolate	35% Sugar by Volume
Milk Chocolate	55% Sugar by Volume

While there are other chocolates available, these are the most commonly used chocolates used in desserts. Knowing their sugar volume can help you to better determine what desserts should land on your plate, and which ones you should avoid.

Dessert Portions Cheat Sheet	
Type of Food	**Serving Size**
Dried Fruit	¼ cup
Pie	1 piece equivalent to the size of a 40-watt light bulb

| Cake | 1 piece that is 1" wide x 2" tall |

Try Fruit Based Desserts

Fruit based desserts will contain dramatically less calories than a sweetened dessert, such as chocolate cake. You can also reduce the calories that are contained in your dessert by using natural sweeteners to create them. Using raw sugar in your desserts can dramatically reduce the amount of calories in your dessert, as can using raw fruits to start your dessert.

ACTION PLAN

Enjoying dessert is one way to indulge without over indulging. In order to ensure that you are successful in obtaining your weight loss goals, utilize negative calorie snacks throughout the day to save up calories for your dessert. Even more important than what your dessert contains, is the serving size. Make sure to stick to adequate serving sizes when you are ordering your dessert.

Everyday Habit #29

The Easiest Alternative to Working Out

Walking is great exercise, and for many, the results are much better than running. Not only is walking great for losing weight, but it is also great for loosening up your joints and making yourself feel lighter after a meal. Walking briskly obviously burns more calories than walking slowly. However, the exact number of calories varies depending on your weight and the rate that you walk. The more you weigh, the more calories you will burn in each walk.

You should make it a habit to walk for at least 30 minutes per day, seven days per week. This will ensure that you keep up with your weight loss goals, your fitness goals, and that you keep yourself in the habit of walking daily. As you time your walk, you will notice that you get farther and farther in the 30 minutes you have allotted. You will also notice that your pants get a looser, little by little.

Why Walking is better than Running

Walking is a lot less damaging to your joints. It also allows you to lose weight at a steadier pace. Also, if you set a goal to walk every day, you are more likely to stick to your goals than if you try to convince yourself to begin running every day when you are just starting out.

As you see the weight melt away and you become more confident in your ability to maintain an exercise program, you can begin jogging and eventually running. Just take your exercise goals slow and pace yourself. Do not take on more than you are comfortable taking on at one time.

Lower Your Cholesterol

Walking helps to increase your good cholesterol and lower bad cholesterol. Managing a balanced cholesterol level can help to reduce the chances of you building up plaque in your arteries, as well as prevents your body from storing fat in problem areas.

Build Up Your Endurance

By building your endurance you are strengthening your cardiovascular system as well as reducing gasses from your body that are considered toxic, and increasing the amount of oxygen your cells are getting. This ensures that your body works efficiently in many different ways, including digestion.

Fat Burning

The average person walks at approximately three miles per hour. If you walk at the average pace of three miles per hour for at least 30 minutes, you will have burned 140 calories. By doing this daily, you will have accomplished burning 980 calories per week. The calculations in the example above are completed taking into consideration that you are already within a normal BMI or body mass index, for your body type. However, if you are heavier, you can burn dramatically more each time you walk because you are carrying more weight and more resistance.

Feeling Better in General

Not only will you burn fat, you can also improve your overall mood by walking daily. Walking relieves stress and can allow your body to reduce negative chemicals in your brain that reduce the mood you feel. It is important for you to relax your mind during this walk, as it can reduce the effects of depression, as well as improve your overall mood for the rest of the day.

ACTION PLAN

Even if you are not yet ready to walk for a full 30 minutes per day, you can still get out there and walk. Even 10 minutes a day is better than sitting around packing on the pounds. Slowly work your way up to 30 minutes per day of walking. Once you reach 30 minutes of walking comfortably, you can increase your walking time, or even your walking pace.

Make sure to stay hydrated while you are walking to maximize the fat burning potential of every trip. Use walking to improve your mood whenever you need. If at any point you feel down, depressed, or as though you need to eat when you are not hungry, taking a walk can increase your chances of overcoming feelings that you do not wish to experience.

Everyday Habit #30

Binge Drink on Water!

Drinking eight glasses of water may seem impossible to some, but only until you really try it will you see that it's not hard at all. Eight glasses of water should total 64 ounces. So, we are not referring to the large "tumbler" style glasses that most people are used to seeing in their cabinets.

The recommended 64 ounces of water is the amount of water necessary to stay fully hydrated and fully energized, which plays a huge role in losing weight and keeping it off. It also plays a huge role in feeling better about yourself and developing balanced health.

A body that is fully hydrated is able to get rid of waste and process out impurities faster. It is also able to burn fat faster. If you are wondering how drinking water will help you lose weight, what we have to say next will fascinate you.

The Role of Water in Weight Loss

No matter how much fat you burn, if it has no way out of your body, it never really leaves. The only way for the fat you burn to exit your body is through your blood stream and through one of the three main exit paths that your body has set up to process it. Your body can burn fat as fuel, especially if you are working out rigorously. Body fat produces energy faster than stored carbohydrates, but it can only be used as fuel if you are fully hydrated.

The second method that your body has is to bring the fat to the skin's surface. It does this through the blood stream. The fat is brought to the skin's surface through capillaries; it is then pushed through your skin with sweat while you are working out.

The third method is through elimination. However, if you are not fully hydrated, the fat that you burn will not make it this far. Without enough water in your body, your digestive system may not be able to carry it all the way to an exit point, which means it will be deposited somewhere else in your body.

This is why problem areas, like the stomach, hips and thighs exist. These are the easiest places for your body to deposit fat, where it cannot bother anything important besides your self-image.

As an added benefit, you will gain more energy and crave less of the unhealthy drinks that once controlled your life.

ACTION PLAN

Don't jump into drinking 8 glasses of water per day. Slowly increase the amount of water you drink each day so that you develop this new habit comfortably and effectively.

Once your plan is in action, keep it in motion. At first, you may feel uncomfortable as your body adjusts to the change. Make sure to give yourself time to really feel the benefits of this change. You will develop more energy and feel more balanced after you have adjusted to your new habit.

If you absolutely do not like water, or you completely detest drinking something without flavor, choose a sugar free water flavoring to add to your water. Pick flavors that you like and keep the amount of flavoring that you add light to reduce the number of calories that you take in. It is important to ensure that you pay attention to the number of calories that you are adding to your water if the flavoring is sweetened or contains artificial sweetener. These calories should be counted into your daily calorie count.

Everyday Habit #31

Reduce Refined Sugars in Your Diet

Refined sugars are found in a wide variety of products. Most of the products that you think of when referring to "refined sugar" products are junk food. But did you know that refined sugars can be found in a wide variety of products that most people see as healthy? Even table sugar is considered a refined sugar, because it is not in its raw form.

Sugar that is in its raw form is actually very healthy for you, but is not extremely sweet. The only sugar that you should have in your diet is natural sugar or sugar cane. While they are not as sweet as refined sugars, it is definitely better for you than the alternative.

How Sugar Causes Weight Gain

Sugar causes weight gain because your body must break it down or store it somewhere. If your body cannot break it down, it stores it for later use inside fat cells. The more you feed fat cells, the faster they can duplicate, which leads to weight gain.

Sugar Causes Insulin Resistance

This is not something you should ignore, even if you are not diabetic. Eating sugar on a regular basis makes your body more immune to its presence.

Once your body becomes used to the idea of having a high higher than usual blood sugar, it begins to ignore the levels inside of your body. This can lead to weight gain and eventually diabetes or a pre-diabetic state.

Refined Sugar is a Simple Carbohydrate

Refined sugar is a simple carbohydrate. Refined sugars are found mostly in foods that are processed and are unhealthy for you. These sugars distract your digestive system from deriving any nutrition from the other food you eat and cause sudden increases in your blood sugar.

If your body is not able to produce enough insulin at once to break down the sugar and flush it from your body, it is stored as fat in your body.

Sugar is Empty Calories

Refined sugars provide no nutritional value, but they do provide empty calories for your body. Many people do not count these calories into their daily calorie count, so it is very easy for you to go over your desired calorie count, which causes extra weight gain.

ACTION PLAN

It is important that you avoid as many products as possible that contain refined sugars. This will help you to reduce unexpected calories and compensate for those that you do take in.

Avoid foods that are processed, such as snack cakes, chips, soda and other foods that are considered "junk food." If you do choose eat or drink these products make sure to count them into your daily calorie count so you can compensate for them.

You will also need to take into account how many carbohydrates are in the food or beverage as well, because processed carbohydrates do not process the same as whole grain carbohydrates.

Everyday Habit #32

The Wonders of a Single Cup of Green Tea Daily

Not only is green tea relaxing, it also has tremendous weight loss benefits. Green tea contains ingredients that are effective on a biological level. These ingredients not only make you healthier, but they also increase your ability to lose weight.

Green tea contains caffeine. The level of caffeine that it contains is about half of what you would receive from a cup of coffee. While it does not have a high amount of caffeine, there is still enough to create a mild effect.

Caffeine is a stimulant that aids in fat burning. The ingredients that you are aiming for with weight loss effects, and mood enhancement, are actually the antioxidants that green tea contains. The antioxidants that it contains are considered catechins. These antioxidants can help boost metabolism, break down fat, and aid in transporting fat cells to the "exit points" of the body.

Green tea also contains a specific antioxidant called norepinephrine. This is an enzyme that is created inside the body. Its purpose is to stimulate the nervous system to stimulate fat cells to break down.

Combining Green Tea with Exercise

When combined with exercise, consuming green tea daily can help to increase the rate that fat is burned during exercise. So, while green tea help burn fat while you are at rest, the effects can be increased dramatically if you use it in combination with a regular exercise program.

Don't Like Drinking Green Tea? Try a Supplement!

If you do not like drinking green tea, you can easily find a supplement that provides the same benefits, but in tablet or capsule form. These supplements provide a concentrated form of green tea and it gives all of the benefits in a small package that can be taken once to three times per day.

Shop around and find supplements that are made with quality ingredients that are made by reputable companies and have been tested by independent laboratories for quality and purity standards. The best green tea supplements are not always expensive, but certified supplements will not be found at a cheap price.

In order to find one that provides health benefits, weight loss, balance and safety will require a little research on your part, but is well worth the effort you put into the search.

ACTION PLAN

Drinking a cup of green tea daily can help to increase the amount of fat burned while at rest and can increase the amount of fat burned while exercising.

As an addition, drinking green tea daily can help you to feel more energized and refreshed. It helps to cleanse the body of impurities. To get the maximum benefit from green tea, drink one to two cups of it every day. If you have an exercise regimen, drink it about one to two hours before you begin your workout.

Make sure that any green tea supplement you choose does not interact with medications that you are currently taking. If you have health conditions that limit the amount of caffeine that you can take in on a daily basis, you may want to avoid green tea products as they can increase your heart rate and do not always mix well with medications that are used to treat heart conditions. Just like with any other supplement, you should check with your doctor to ensure that you are healthy enough to withstand the increased heart rate that you may experience.

Never take green tea supplements in the evening, as they contain a lot of caffeine and they can keep you awake at night. If you find that taking the supplement in the afternoon causes sleepless nights, or makes sleeping difficult, only take the supplement in the morning.

Everyday Habit #33

Don't Ditch Breakfast

One of the major mistakes that dieters make is to skip breakfast. They think that if they avoid the extra calories, they can lose weight faster. However, eating a healthy breakfast can actually help you lose weight, while skipping breakfast in the morning can cause you to gain weight. Strangely, it can cause you to gain weight faster than eating an unhealthy diet

By skipping breakfast in the morning, your body craves higher calorie foods in the afternoon hours. These are the foods that make you gain weight. Studies have proven that those who skip breakfast are more likely to give into the cravings they feel for higher calorie foods.

The Brain's Response to Fasting

When you make a habit of fasting, or skipping breakfast in an effort to lose weight, your body begins to store fat because it is naturally inclined to do so. This is because your body can survive off of the fat that is stored away for later use. Essentially, by skipping breakfast, you are convincing your body that food is in short supply, which increases the amount of fat that it feels the need to store in your body for later survival.

Who knew that skipping breakfast could send your body into survival mode? Your body will continue to store fat until it realizes that food is not in short supply, which can take a day, or up to a week to reset. So, skipping one breakfast can set your diet back by ten or more pounds!

ACTION PLAN

By simply eating a healthy breakfast every morning, you can reduce the amount of weight you gain. Choosing foods that are high in fiber and healthy carbohydrates can greatly reduce the amount of fat that your body stores. Eat foods like oatmeal, fruits, or whole grain cereal in the morning to give yourself a boost of energy and to prevent the amount of fat your body stores from later meals. If you are in hurry, something as simple as a whole grain bagel can provide the nutritional value that your body needs to make it through until lunch. With a breakfast that simple, there is no reason to skip such an important meal.

Everyday Habit #34

Sleep Enough!

So how can sleep help you lose weight? Sleep controls more than just your everyday energy levels and you will be amazed at what getting between six to eight hours of sleep can do for your body.

Reducing the Amount You Eat

Getting six to eight hours of sleep each night helps regulate the amount of leptin that your body creates. Leptin is the hormone that helps your body realize when you have eaten enough. Failing to get enough sleep can decrease the amount of leptin your body creates, which causes you to overeat. Getting enough sleep also helps to regulate the amount of ghrelin that your body releases. This hormone helps to stimulate your appetite and tells you when you are hungry.

Reducing Stress and Anxiety

Stress and anxiety are two main contributors in why your body deposits fat around your midsection. Getting between six to eight hours of sleep per night can greatly reduce anxiety and stress, which lead to belly fat.

Sleeping Too Much

Sleeping too much can have the opposite effect on your body. Sleeping for more than nine hours at a time can cause your body to fast for too long, putting it into survival mode, similar to if you were to skip breakfast repeatedly.

ACTION PLAN

Arrange your schedule in a way that allows you to get between six to eight hours of sleep per night. Having a regular sleeping schedule is important to ensure that you get an adequate amount of sleep without overdoing it. If you find that no matter what you do, you cannot sleep 8 hours per night, you should speak to your doctor.

Do not sleep more than nine hours per night. This can actually have the opposite effect on your body and cause you to be overly tired and feel drained. It can also cause you to ingest additional calories during the day from caffeinated beverages that contain empty calories.

If you find that you are sleeping more than nine hours per night, you should contact your doctor. This could mean that you have an underlying health problem that you are not aware of and could be serious. Your doctor can determine whether your abnormal sleep patterns are due to a vitamin deficiency, a stressful life, or other factors that are talking a toll on your health.

Everyday Habit #35

Eat Colorful Meals

The old adage that claiming that the more colorful your meal is, the better it is for you is actually true. Try to combine a wide array of vegetables on your plate at every meal.

Not only will this make the less desirable part of your meal more appealing, but it will also round out the amount of calories that you get at every meal. By eating colorful meals, you are adding in lower calorie vegetables and a wider variety of nutrients to your diet.

So what is the Real Trick?

Foods that are vibrant in color provide more nutrients and are natural sources of vitamins and nutrients. By eating more natural foods, you are avoiding processed foods, which cause you to put on pounds faster than you normally would. Colorful meals ensure that you are eating healthy!

Mixing Your Vegetables

Some frozen vegetables can be purchased pre-mixed. However, if you have specific vegetables that you like to mix together, that is great! If you are not sure what vegetables you like mixed, the only way to figure it out is through trial and error. Mix and match various vegetables on a regular basis to ensure that you get a well-rounded, balanced nutrient base in your diet.

ACTION PLAN

Evaluate the color of the meals you eat now. Are they bright, vibrant and exciting colors? If not, chances are you are not getting enough vitamins and nutrients in your current meals. Plan meals that are vibrant in color every day. If you are not the biggest fan of vegetables, experiment with different cooking methods to determine how you like them best. Each cooking method yields a different flavor. Don't like them cooked? Toss these vegetables into a salad and see if you feel different about them in a raw state.

Everyday Habit #36

Eat Negative Calorie Snack Foods

Did you know that there are negative calorie foods out there that won't cause you to gain weight? Well, there are plenty of them. Most of the foods that are considered negative calorie are found in the fresh produce section of your local grocery store. Fresh produce items that are not considered starches contain less calories than it takes to chew and digest. This means that you can fill yourself up on them periodically throughout the day without worrying that you will gain weight. This makes them the perfect snack food.

Best Negative Calorie Snack Foods

The best negative calorie snack foods that you can stock up on are:

- Asparagus
- Broccoli
- Cauliflower

- Celery
- Cucumbers
- Garlic
- Green beans
- Green cabbage
- Iceberg lettuce
- Onions
- Radishes
- Spinach
- Turnips

The more negative calorie foods you eat every day, the less empty calories you will consume on a regular basis. This allows you to control your calorie intake and ensure that most of your calorie intake comes from the meals that you have planned beforehand.

ACTION PLAN

Enjoy these low-calorie snacks between meals. To add extra nutritional value to your snack, add in a handful of nuts to your snack. The added protein will provide a great energy boost. You can also mix low calorie vegetables in with starchy vegetables to ensure balance out your meal, make it more filling without adding a ton of calories to your meal. It is also a great way to balance out high calorie starches that are in the rest of your meal.

Everyday Habit #37

Consume Healthy Fats Regularly

While scientists are screaming that fat is bad for you, the truth is that not all fat is bad. Healthy fats do exist and are necessary for you to lose weight and to gain muscle. Healthy fats are considered unsaturated fats, which are essentially fats that do not solidify in your arteries. There are many fats and oils that are considered unsaturated and most of these fats come from vegetable-based sources and from fish. Eating a healthy amount of unsaturated fat everyday can increase the amount of weight you lose on a regular basis. The most popular fat right now comes from a product called coconut oil. This oil is pressed from freshly picked coconuts and can be used to cook with and added to everyday drinks, like coffee or tea.

Choose Meat that are Lean

Meats that are lean should be your primary focus. Meats like chicken and fish are better for you than red meat. This is because the fat that is contained in red meat is harder for the body to process and cannot be used as effectively as fuel. This makes it more likely that your body will store the fat that is contained in red meat for later use, and process the fat that is contained in leaner meats.

If you do eat red meat on a regular basis, or even on occasion, ensure that the meat is as lean as possible. For example, choose 80/20 hamburger meat over 70/30 hamburger meat. While 10% less fat may not seem like much, it can make a dramatic difference in the way your body digests the fat, and how much fat it stores from your meal.

ACTION PLAN

Add at least two teaspoons of healthy fat to every meal you eat. It is easy to do this by sautéing your vegetables in coconut or soybean oils. Change your healthy oils on a regular basis and according to what you are cooking. As we have mentioned before, each oil has its own use, as well as its own temperature yield. Some are good for baking, others are good for frying, and yet others are good for sautéing.

Everyday Habit #38

Create Your Own Flavored Water

If you do not like to drink regular water, want to kick your soda addiction, or you are looking for a better way to enjoy water, creating your own flavored water can help you increase your water intake each day. How do you create your own flavored water? Simply cut up pieces of your favorite fruits and place them in a pitcher of water. Allow it to sit for 24 hours in the refrigerator to allow the flavor from the fruit to release into the water. Not only will you enjoy this water more, you will save money on those expensive flavored water drinks and there are no added artificial sweeteners. There is no need to strain the fruit from the water; it will provide you something to chew on while you enjoy your water.

How Does This Help You Lose Weight?

Creating your own flavored water doesn't just make your water taste better, but it will increase the amount of water you drink on a daily basis. It also provides natural sugars that can keep your body running at top speed throughout the day. It is also a great way to sneak fruit into your diet without having to count servings on a daily basis.

It Tastes Great!

We all love adding flavoring to our water because water doesn't have much of a flavor on its own. This is why we are tempted to lean more toward sodas, flavored seltzer waters, and artificially sweetened drinks. By creating a naturally flavored drink with a natural sweetener, you are less likely to indulge in sodas or artificially sweetened juices.

Create Your Own "Soda"

Creating your own soda is not as difficult as it sounds. Simply purchase unsweetened seltzer water and cut pieces of fruit into small enough pieces to fit inside the bottle. Reseal the bottle and allow it to sit in the refrigerator overnight.

ACTION PLAN

Make it a habit to drink water on a daily basis. In order to ensure that your body is fully hydrated, you should take in at least 64 ounces of water per day. By adding bits of fruit to it, you are making it more enjoyable to drink this water and add some excitement to your daily routine. Simply cut up several servings of your favorite fruit and place it in a pitcher of water. Allow the water to sit in the refrigerator for 24 hours to allow the vitamins to fuse into the water.

Feel daring? Mix several types of fruit together to create your own flavor mixtures. The best fruits to mix if you want to lose weight are citrus fruits. This is because they provide added acidity and can help to break down fat. Citrus fruits help to balance your body's pH, which can dramatically improve your health and wellness, as well as balance your weight in a healthy way.

Everyday Habit #39

Strength Training Boosts Fat Loss!

Strength training on a regular basis builds muscle. The more muscle density you have, the easier it is to lose weight. While this may sound like you must complete an intense workout, strength training is anything that builds strength and stamina. Does the thought of strength training bother you? It is probably because lifting heavy weights may not be for you. However, strength training does not always include lifting a lot of weight. Simply starting with three-pound weights and lifting them in various ways on a daily basis can help you to build muscle slowly and build your endurance. Simple exercises, like squats, walking and lifting light weights can increase the amount of fat you burn and can increase the amount of muscle you build underneath the unwanted weight.

Once you have successfully began building muscle, you will notice that the excess weight you carry will melt away faster through using the other tips in this book.

ACTION PLAN

It doesn't matter if the weights you lift are three pounds or fifty pounds, you are still building muscle by lifting them on a regular basis. When combined with regular exercise and a great diet, you will lose weight faster than you would expect. The more muscle density you have from lifting weights, the easier it is for your body to burn fat, so focusing on building muscle can increase your chances of reaching your weight loss and health goals in a shorter period of time.

Everyday Habit #40

This Habit Will Make You Eat LESS

By making plates at the stove, you can control portion sizes and resist the urge to take seconds on the unhealthier portion of your dinner. Making plates at the table allows you to limit portion sizes, measure foods that you feel are important to be accurate on, and ensures that you are eating healthy portions of each food. Making your plate at the table, and keeping the serving bowls at the table makes it easier to over indulge in foods and can cause you to eat faster in order to enjoy more of the foods you like.

Do Not Allow Your Eyes to Become Bigger than Your Belly

Your stomach can only hold 4 cups of food before it reaches the point where it has stretched too far for comfort. Carefully monitor the amount of food that you put on your plate. Keep serving sizes in mind when you are plating your food and make sure that you take into account that a child's stomach is half the size of an adult's, so they should be served half as much. A toddler will only need ¼ the amount of an adult.

Children and Proteins

Very young children do not gravitate toward proteins, especially if they are meat based. You may need to provide a vegetable or soy-based protein in place of the meat-based protein that you typically offer to older children. Keep soy-based proteins on hand if you have a child who does not like the texture of meat or does not like specific types of meat.

Unless you are a vegetarian, offer meat-based protein first and encourage your child to eat it. If you cannot accomplish getting them to eat the meat-based protein, either through flat out refusal, or through refusal of texture, offer a soy-based protein in its place. Since the texture and weight is different, they will be more likely to accept the soy-based protein.

ACTION PLAN

Making your plate at the stove makes it easier for you to follow the basic plating rules. Half of your plate should consist of vegetables and the other half of your plate should be divided in half, between your protein and your carbohydrate.

Everyday Habit #41

Break Your Weight Loss Goals into Manageable Pieces

So, you want to lose 50 pounds? Well, losing 50 pounds is a great goal, but does it really give you much to look forward to? Unless you lose all 50 pounds, you don't reach your goal, which can be depressing and can cause you to give up before you even get near your goal.

Breaking your weight loss goals down into more manageable pieces can be vital to reaching your goals. For example, saying, "I want to lose one pound 50 times" gives you 50 reasons to celebrate instead of one single goal.

ACTION PLAN

Break your weight loss goals down into manageable pieces so that you can reward yourself for reaching a goal. The more manageable each goal is, the easier it is to obtain and the less time you have to wait until you reach your goal.

Everyday Habit #42

Pack Your Lunch

When you are working, it is so easy to grab something to eat from the sandwich shop around the corner. While this is simple and easy to do, it is also not healthy since you do not know what preservatives they use in their food, and you cannot ensure that the foods that they are serving are full of unhealthy fillers.

Packing a healthy lunch that is all-natural and well-balanced can help you control the foods that go into your body on a daily basis. It gives you the same control that you have at home, which allows you to stick to your meal plan and can help remove excuses that may arise while you are on your journey to eating healthier.

Don't Forget to Pack Snacks

While that vending machine on the third floor looks appealing, you should stay away at all costs. By packing your own snacks, you no longer have an excuse to visit the machine if hunger strikes. Packing foods that are considered negative calories, nuts, and no-sugar-added dry fruit, can help satisfy cravings - helping you maintain your weight goals.

ACTION PLAN

When you are creating your meal plan for your breakfast and dinner meals, make sure to include healthy choices for lunch. Planning to pack your lunch and snacks can greatly reduce the urge to make unhealthy choices that you will regret later and will pack on pounds that you are trying to avoid.

Everyday Habit #43

Use Smaller Plates

While purchasing plates was not on the top of your list of ways to lose weight, it can definitely help you to reduce the amount you eat at each meal. Science proves that you eat with your eyes before you sit down to eat. Your brain tells you that in order to fill up at dinner, your plate should be full. By using a smaller plate, you trick your brain into thinking you ate more than you really did.

The Same Plating Rule Remains

Even if you are using smaller plate you should still separate it in the same way you would a larger plate. One half of your plate should be filled with vegetables, and the other half should be evenly split between meat and carbohydrate servings. This ensures that you are still getting healthy portions of each main element in your diet.

Choose Red Plates

While you may not have considered the color of your plates as a method of losing weight, many scientific studies have shown that eating your meals off of a red plate will actually reduce the amount of food you eat at a single setting.

ACTION PLAN

If you are currently using 12-inch dinner plates, purchase 10-inch dinner plates. While this difference may not sound like a lot, it can make a dramatic difference in the amount that you eat on a regular basis. Purchase dinner plates that are red, or a variation of red to comfortably reduce the amount you eat on a regular basis.

Everyday Habit #44

Reduce or Remove Red Meat from Your Diet

Red meat contains a higher concentration of saturated fat, as well as fat that is difficult for your body to digest. This is why the texture of red meat is so different from the texture of chicken or fish. If your body does manage to break down the fat that is contained in red meat, it can easily become a stored fat in your body, since your digestives system is not sure what to do with it or how to use it.

There are hundreds of other health reasons to avoid red meat that do not pertain directly to weight loss that will make your stomach turn, but that is not our main focus.

Red Meat Leads to Obesity

There are several studies that have proven a direct correlation between the consumption of red meat and obesity. These studies also showed that the more often you eat red meat, the more likely you are to gain weight and keep it on. Even if you do not plan to remove red meat from your diet completely, you should at least reduce it to a once a week indulgence and monitor the amount of red meat you do eat.

ACTION PLAN

The average serving size for any type of red meat is about the size of a deck of cards, or about 4 ounces. Making sure that you only put red meat on the menu once per week can dramatically reduce the amount of stubborn weight gain that you experience.

Everyday Habit #45

Eat Slower

A well-known scientific fact has shown that it takes 20 minutes for your body to realize that it is full. It also takes an average of three minutes for the food you just swallowed to make it to your stomach. Unless you give your body time to register that it is full, you may have just eaten twice as much as your body needs to actually feel full.

By eating slower and chewing each bite 10 to 20 times, you are giving your body time to register how it feels and how much food it has taken in. A great way of giving your body time to register what it has eaten is to take a sip of water between each bite. This allows a break in the movement of your fork, but still gives you something to do with your hands while you wait for time for the next bite.

ACTION PLAN

Take your time while eating to ensure that you are not eating more than you really need to. Give your body time to register whether or not you feel full before you think of taking seconds on food. Never speed-eat! Always take your time while eating to ensure that you are not consuming any unnecessary calories. If this means sitting down at a table to eat, then do it.

Everyday Habit #46

Snack on Vegetables and Nuts

Vegetables and nuts are a great snack food, but for different reasons.

Vegetables

Many vegetables provide negative calories, which means that they take burn more calories while you are chewing and digesting than they actually contain.

Vegetables also take a long time to chew, which gives you plenty of time to register whether you have reached the point of satisfaction.

Nuts

Nuts make a great snack food. They are crunchy, slightly salty (if you choose) and provide a lot of protein. Protein can help increase energy and fill you up better than anything you can find in a vending machine or drive through.

ACTION PLAN

Make sure to keep nuts and vegetables readily available. Pack vegetables and nuts for road trips as well as snacks at the office. Keeping nuts around the house can help keep you from indulging in junk food that may be hidden in the pantry, or over indulging in leftovers that are packed with carbohydrates that are tempting you in the fridge.

Everyday Habit #47

Meditate Daily

Meditation is a great way to become aware of your body and what you feel. Since stress is a main contributor to weight gain, daily mediation can help to reduce stress and allow you to learn how to pay attention to the cues that your body gives you on a regular basis.

Once you have determined what signals your body sends you at various times of the day, you can make the right choices to suit the needs of your body.

While stress is a major contributing factor in weight gain, not understanding what your body is telling you is another contributing factor. If you are hungry, if you are thirsty, if you are just frustrated, you may not be able to tell the difference in the cues your body is sending you, which can cause you to eat when it is not necessary.

Becoming more aware of your body can help you determine the difference between hunger and thirst, as well as whether your body is requesting food in response to stress.

ACTION PLAN

Meditate daily by following these simple instructions.

1. Sit in a comfortable, quite place that is free from distractions
2. Close your eyes and relax your muscles
3. Breathe deeply and slowly
4. Clear your mind completely and pay attention to what your body feels at every moment.

By meditating during episodes of hunger that are uncharacteristic of your typical daily routine, you can decipher whether your body is really telling you that it is hungry, or whether your body is telling you something else.

Everyday Habit #48

Avoid Artificial Sweeteners

While many companies like to pretend that artificial sweeteners are better for you, the truth is that they can cause you to gain weight faster than natural sugars and they can contribute to the development of cancer.

Using Pure Sugar Products

If you plan to use a sugar product in your meals or your drinks, choose raw sugar products over processed or artificial versions. Raw sugar is not the same as table sugar. Many people are not aware that the white sugar they keep in their cabinets, commonly referred to as "table sugar" us actually a processed sugar product and leads to the development of diabetes and insulin resistance. While raw sugar products can cause you to gain some weight over time, they do not have as much of an impact on your weight as processed sugar or artificial sweeteners.

Safe Sweeteners

If you plan to use sweeteners in your food or drink, choose a raw sugar product, or honey. These products add a great sweet flavor without going overboard.

ACTION PLAN

Keep processed sugar products and artificial sweeteners out of your pantry. If they are present, you will be more tempted to use them. Always keep raw sugar products and honey on hand in the case that you may need to use a sweetener. Avoid any product that is not openly made of real sugar. Research how each product is modified to determine whether the sugar was processed, chemicals were added, fillers were added, or there are any precautions you should take when using the sweetener.

Everyday Habit #49

Replace One Meal a Day with a Protein Shake

Protein shakes are a great way to ensure that you are getting the proper amount of vitamins and minerals. One of the main ways to ensure that you are eating a diet that will help you lose weight is to balance your protein, fat and carbohydrate intake with your vegetable intake. Other than carbohydrates, protein is the most important substance to take in every day. Without it, your body does not have the building blocks that it needs to create muscle, or repair tissue that has been damaged through daily activity.

Protein shakes typically contain a well-balanced amount of protein, fat and carbohydrates, which ensures that you are getting an adequate "meal" even though it is in a liquid form. Since this "meal" is in a liquid form, your body is able to absorb the nutrients from the shake without straining or without having to go through a difficult digestive process. Protein shakes contain fewer calories than a traditional meal would.

Talk to Your Doctor

Before you begin starting a regimen that involves replacing a meal with a protein shake, make sure to talk to your doctor for safety reasons. Some health conditions may prevent you from being able to make this change, while others may simply require you to eat a low-calorie snack while you are enjoying your shake. For some people, starting a protein shake regimen can cause an upset stomach and a little bit of a queasy feeling.

ACTION PLAN

The best way to ensure that you are successful in achieving weight loss through protein shake meal replacement is to replace only one meal per day with a high-quality protein shake that has been reinforced with vitamins and nutrients. There are many inexpensive protein-based shakes that are available at your local supermarket that will serve the purpose of supplementing your diet.

If you prefer to purchase more specific, or more potent, protein shakes, you can do so online or through your local nutrition supplementation store.

Everyday Habit #50

Take a Multi-Vitamin Daily

Many hunger cues are caused by your body lacking essential vitamins and nutrients, not because you actually need a meal or snack. By adding a quality multi-vitamin to your daily regimen, you can decrease the number of times that your body triggers a hunger cue due to your body being low on a specific vitamin.

Seeking Medical Intervention

If you notice that you are hungry often, or that you crave a certain type of food on a regular basis, you may want to check with your doctor to determine whether you have a specific vitamin deficiency that needs to be treated medically. There are thousands of people throughout the world that suffer from deficiencies in more than one vitamin and a multi-vitamin does not always have an adequate amount of all vitamins for everyone out there, even if it is a high-quality supplement.

Balancing Your Vitamin Intake

Balancing your daily vitamin intake can help you to ensure that you do not over eat, or eat when it isn't necessary, which can directly relate to the weight gain you have experienced in the past. By balancing your vitamin intake, you can reduce the amount of food you take in on a daily basis, which can translate into weight loss, especially if you exercise and take a protein supplement as well.

ACTION PLAN

A quality multi-vitamin does not come at a discount price. Most quality multi-vitamins are not cheap but there are some things that you should take into consideration before purchasing any multi-vitamin.

1. Just because a multi-vitamin is expensive doesn't mean it is effective.
2. Research the product before you make a purchase.
3. Make sure that the company that created the product is known for producing quality products.
4. Ensure that the product has been tested by an independent party.
5. Always check with your doctor to determine if whether you have a sensitivity or allergy to specific vitamins or minerals.

Once again, thank you for reading this book, and I hope you're getting a lot of valuable information. I would greatly appreciate it if you could take 30 seconds to leave me a review for this book on Amazon.com.

Everyday Habit #51

Don't Forget Fish

While you should always provide variety in your diet, scientific research shows that eating low fat, white fish at least two to three times per week can help you lose weight and manage your weight more effectively than other diets.

Eat Fish High in Omega 3 Two to Three Times for Week

By eating fish that is high in Omega 3 on a regular basis, you can help control your weight, increase your energy and increase muscle mass. It is important that you choose the fish that you eat carefully. You should only eat wild caught fish, as they contain a higher amount of omega 3 fatty acids because of the diet they survive off of in the wild. Farm raised fish tend to have less omega 3 and a higher saturated fat content due to the diet they are forced to eat.

Types of Fish to Eat

Black cod or sable fish – and sable fish is a great source of omega 3 fatty acids. They are also rich in selenium, which is known to assist in weight loss and provide essential nutrients to growing muscle.

Halibut – One serving of halibut contains enough omega 3 fatty acid to count as one day's serving. Halibut is also a great source of B12, which is essential for heart health and blood flow.

Sardines, herring and anchovies – All three of these fish are high in omega 3 fatty acids. While it is preferred that you eat fresh fish, canned fish can easily be incorporated into your diet for convenient meals.

ACTION PLAN

When planning your weekly meals, incorporate fish into your diet at least twice per week. When shopping, make sure to look for white fish that specifically states that it is a wild caught fish product. It is recommended for you to eat fish in as fresh of a form as possible. While canned fish can be substituted for fresh fish, the quality of the fish is not as high as it would have been if the fish were fresh.

Everyday Habit #52

Avoid Places You Used to Eat At

If you are used to eating at certain restaurants and you are known for making bad food choices at these places, avoid them at all costs.

The purpose of creating new habits must start from a place that is fresh in your own mind. Choose restaurants with healthier choices and make daring decisions from the menu. Before going out to eat, develop a clear idea of what you will order and how you will order it. This will prevent you from making a comfortable choice off of the menu that does not provide the health benefits you are looking for.

Beginning Again

Once you have developed the ability to make proper food choices, you can once again go to the restaurants that you used to frequent. You will be able to make decisions based on the new experiences you have learned through experiencing other settings.

Avoid Fast Food

Fast food is unhealthy for your body - period. It is full of preservatives and byproducts that your body should not be exposed to in any way. These byproducts can cause excessive, rapid weight gain. The preservatives that are found in fast food can also cause serious weight gain as well as water retention.

ACTION PLAN

Just because you are trying to lose weight, does not mean that you cannot eat out, it simply means that you must make smarter food choices. Many restaurants have low fat or low-calorie menu items, and some even have menus that are aimed at specific diets or avoiding specific foods that cause allergic reactions or weight gain. Many restaurants have their menus listed online, with nutritional facts. This can help you to make your decision based on your personal dietary needs and your weight loss goals.

Everyday Habit #53

Avoid Empty Liquid Calories

Most of the beverages we drink on a daily basis contain empty calories. Drinks like coffee (depending on how you have it), dark teas, sodas, artificial fruit juices and flavored drinks that contain artificial sweeteners can add a lot of calories to your diet.

Many people who have struggled for years to lose weight have seen firsthand that changing what they drink can have a dramatic effect on their current weight. There are countless, true stories that can be easily accessed online that will explain how simply cutting out soda from their daily diet allowed people to lose over 100 pounds in a matter of a year. This is a significant impact!

Carefully Analyze Your Liquid Calories

Most people count the calories that they eat on a daily basis, but they tend to ignore the calories that they drink. Because of this, you could have several hundred extra calories that are unaccounted for. While it sounds small, these uncounted calories can cause you to develop extra weight gain because you do not know that these calories need to be burned.

Diabetics and Soda

If you have diabetes and you drink soda on a regular basis, even if it is diet, you could begin gaining weight at a very rapid pace. This is because your body is not able to process out the sugar, or the sugar substitute is not processed out of your body.

For diabetics, the sugar that your body cannot process can easily be stored in your body fat as a way to "tuck it away" where the body does not have to deal with it. Over time, this leads to excess weight gain and insulin resistance which can cause damage to your heart and other organs, as well as risk your life.

ACTION PLAN

Make sure to include all calories that you ingest on a daily basis, even if they are from a liquid source. If you are worried about the calories you are taking in on a regular basis, avoid high calorie liquid sources and focus on drinking water, or water that has been flavored with fruit. If you are at a restaurant, simply squeezing lemon into your water can make it more appealing than a soda.

Everyday Habit #54

Try Yoga

While most people are leaning toward the old adage of cardio being the best way to burn fat and build muscle they are overlooking a better way to achieve the same result. Yoga is a great way to burn fat, build muscle and develop strength and endurance in a low impact setting. If you are not a fan of a rapid heart rate, yoga may be for you.

Yoga is a great way to develop core strength and burn fat without causing injury to your joints. Because of the strength and stability that is needed to hold your body in certain positions, you will burn fat just as fast as you would if you were performing a cardio exercise.

Great for Those Who are Trying to Lose Weight

If you are trying to lose weight, performing cardio exercises can cause excessive wear and tear on your joints as well as extra strain on your tendons and ligaments. The majority of the population is under the impression that you must work up a sweat in order to lose weight. This is not true. The only method of losing weight is to break down fat, which requires building muscle. Even light yoga that involves no sweating and very little straining, can help you lose weight at nearly the same speed as an intense cardio exercise.

Choosing the Right Yoga Poses

Choosing yoga poses that target your specific problem areas is essential to breaking down difficult fat for your personal situation. Since everyone's body is different, everyone develops different problem areas and everyone's body reacts differently to each yoga pose, we cannot specify the specific poses that will help you reach your desired weight or shape.

Each Pose Burns a Different Amount of Calories

Each yoga pose burns fat in different locations and at a different concentration. The more advanced yoga poses you use, the more calories you burn and the more core strength you develop. Work hard to develop your skill level and your core if you plan to lose weight in a fast-paced manner.

ACTION PLAN

Just like with any other exercise plan, you should consult with your doctor before beginning a yoga routine. You should have a full physical examination to ensure that your ligaments, tendons and muscles are strong enough to endure the strength and stamina needed to perform yoga.

If you are unsure of where to begin, you can find yoga classes that suit all needs at pretty much any gym. If you are self-conscious about your abilities, you can sign up for private yoga lessons until you build your self-confidence and your skill level to the point where you are comfortable performing in front of other people in a class.

Everyday Habit #55

Eat Vegetarian Once a Week

By eating vegetarian once a week, you are able to reduce the amount of saturated fat that you take in. It also gives you a great healthy burst of vegetables and carbohydrates for your body to focus on. Scientific studies have proven that eating a vegetarian dinner once per week can help you reduce your weight by ½ to 1 pound per week.

While 1 pound per week may not sound like a lot of weight, think about this amount of weight loss like this. How large is one pound of hamburger meat? When you think about a pound in size instead of weight measurement, it seems a lot better doesn't it?

Make Your Plate as Bright as You Can

While preparing your vegetarian meal, ensure that your plate contains as many types of vegetables and as many colors of vegetables as possible. The brighter your plate is, the more vitamins and minerals it contains.

Choose a Hearty Grain

Typically, if you eat an omnivore-based diet, the meat you ingest keeps you full for a longer duration of time. If you are not used to eating a vegetarian diet, your body may plow through a lightweight carbohydrate in a very short period of time. Choosing a hearty carbohydrate, like bulgur wheat, quinoa, or brown rice will help to ensure that you have a meal that sticks with you for a while.

Keep Negative Calorie Snacks Around on Vegetarian Days

If you are not used to eating a vegetarian based diet, you can keep negative calorie fruits and vegetables around to ensure that if you do get hungry later, you have something to snack on that does not add extra calories to your diet.

Cook Your Vegetables in a Healthy Oil

By cooking your vegetables in healthy oils, like coconut oil, you can help to ensure that your meal is flavorful and healthy. Other oils can be used, such as soybean oil, but do not use oil that contains a high saturated fat content.

Don't Shy Away from Seasoning

When you are seasoning your food, do not be afraid to experiment with various seasonings that you have not tried before. Seasonings like cinnamon, cumin, pepper, red pepper, wasabi and ginger can actually help you lose weight. Seasoning can be your friend and can assist your vegetarian meal in burning fat and giving you the added energy boost your body needs to plow through that excess weight that you are fighting against.

ACTION PLAN

When planning your weekly meals, make sure that you plan one vegetarian meal per week. This meal should contain as many vegetables as possible and should be flavorful and delicious. This will help you to increase your vitamin intake and decrease the amount of saturated fat that you take in each week. Just because there is no meat in your meal does not mean that it has to be boring or free from texture.

Cook your vegetables to al'dente texture to give contrast to your food and ensure that it is pleasing to the palate as well as giving you the sensation of chewing, which can have a direct effect on your sensory system and the feeling of being full.

Everyday Habit #56

Limit Your Sodium Intake

Sodium is contained in pretty much everything that you eat. However, sodium is the main reason why people begin to retain water, which contributes directly to the development of water weight, which can be difficult for you to get rid of unless you know it is the culprit.

By limiting the amount of sodium that you take in every day, you can limit the amount of water weight gain that you experience. The average person should take in no more than 2300 mg of sodium per day, which is actually quite a bit if you eat a healthy diet.

How to Limit Your Sodium Intake

Let's face it, salt makes everything taste better but there are better ways to make your food taste great then using salt alone. There are hundreds of spices and thousands of spice mixtures that can be created to make your food delectable, without adding excess amounts of sodium to your diet.

Learning about Spice Mixtures

Learning about spice mixtures and experimenting with various spices can open a new world of flavor to you and your family. Spices can also make foods that are great for you, but don't suit your personal flavor preferences, more appealing and maybe even change your mind about them.

ACTION PLAN

Hit the Internet and learn about different spice options and how you can combine them to experience a world of flavor that you have neglected throughout your life.

Always introduce one spice at a time into your diet. Spices are a well-known reason for allergic reactions. Because of this, you may want to opt for an allergy test before experimenting with different spices, or introduce them in small quantities with other spices that you have used before.

Everyday Habit #57

Cook Meals at Home When Possible

While going out to eat is great, cooking at home allows you to control the ingredients, the flavor and the fat content of your plate. While trying to lose weight, you should cook your own food as often as possible after researching the nutritional value of each of your ingredients.

There are many websites that are dedicated to developing diet plans around the foods that you like and foods you want to try. Many of these websites can help you create meal plans, snack plans and weight loss goals in measurable increments.

Understanding Your Food

Creating your meals at home allows you to have a better understanding of the nutrition that each meal holds and what vitamins are lacking from your meal. You can also monitor your eating habits so that you know what vitamins you need to supplement on a regular basis, either through multi-vitamins or through isolated vitamins.

Controlling the Type of Cooking Method Used

Controlling the type of cooking method used is just as important as what is on the plate. Ensuring that the nutritional value is maintained through cooking is essential to maintaining a healthy diet that makes you feel great and lose weight.

Controlling the Fat Levels

Controlling the type of fat used in cooking is essential to the nutritional value of the dish. Fats that are natural and vegetable based are ideal, while fruit fats can be just as valuable. Oils like extra virgin olive oil and coconut oil can be used with a lot of versatility in both sweet and savory dishes.

ACTION PLAN

Creating your meal plan and cooking foods at home makes it more likely that you will enjoy your meal, and that you will eat a healthy portion of each of the foods you have chosen to make.

Eating in public and not paying attention to the quantity of food you are eating can cause you to eat more of unhealthy foods that you are trying to avoid. You may also be tempted to focus more on filler foods than healthy foods. By cooking at home, you are taking control of your diet.

Everyday Habit #58

Eat All of Your Meals as a Family

Eating your meals at home, as a family can has been proven to cause you to eat slower. This is because you take your time to talk to the people around you. Eating slower helps your body to experience the full sensation of eating and gives you time to develop the hormones that make you feel full. You are also less likely to feel rushed while eating, which means that you will take your time and eat less.

Eating Meals as a Family Teaches Nutrition

Eating meals as a family teaches your children the value of eating a healthy foods and healthy portions of foods. It also allows you to talk to your children and your spouse, which causes you to eat slower than you typically would. This allows your body time to register the chemicals that your brain creates to cause you to feel full and let you know when it is time to stop eating.

Think About How Much You Should Eat

When you think about how much the average human stomach is meant to hold without becoming distended you will realize how you get that "over stuffed" feeling so easily. The human stomach is meant to hold between 45 and 75 ml of food, or about 4 cups at one time.

While this may sound like a lot of food, this amount of food is what is contained in the stomach when you have that "over stuffed" or "holiday meal" feeling. At this point, the food in your stomach is pushing on your diaphragm and causing discomfort. Until your stomach reaches the point of "full" the hormone ghrelin is not released. However, it takes time for your brain to receive the transmission from your stomach that it has reached a "satisfied" pressure.

By eating slowly, you can give your brain time to register the pressure that your stomach is experiencing to allow you to feel full. If you eat fast, you can easily eat to the point of food pressing against your diaphragm, meaning you are over-full, before your brain realizes that you are even nearing the verge of being full. Sometimes you feel as though you could eat a lot, simply because you feel so hungry. So, keep in mind how much your stomach is meant to hold while making your plate for dinner.

ACTION PLAN

Eating meals as a family has physical health benefits as well as mental health benefits. You can incorporate your children into the cooking experience, which makes them more likely to be daring and eat foods that most children avoid. Eating meals as a family is a great bonding experience and can really help to soothe the soul and the bathroom scale.

Everyday Habit #59

Incorporate Chia Seeds into Your Diet

When most people think of Chia Seeds, they think of a decorative potted plant that grows hair in random places. They also think these devices are just annoying decorations their cat ends up eating before it ever becomes something adorable to look at.

What they don't realize is that Chia Seeds have so much nutritional value and can be added to almost any dish. Not only are they good for you, they also taste great and add amazing texture to your dish.

So How Do Chia Seeds Help You Lose Weight?

Chia seeds can help you lose weight by simply expanding in your stomach as you eat. They are a great filler ingredient that makes you feel as though you have eaten more than you really have.

Many Weight Loss Supplements Contain Chia Seeds

You know those "amazing" weight loss supplements that you simply shake onto your food and it helps to reduce the amount of food you eat? These weight loss supplements are made with chia seeds.

In all actuality, purchasing Chia Seeds from a store shelf can save you a lot of money and take a huge profit away from diet companies that are taking advantage of people who are simply trying to make a positive change in their lives.

Using Chia Seeds to Lose Weight

Chia seeds are a great way to lose weight and are fairly inexpensive. It is recommended that you split 50 grams of Chia seeds daily among your three main meals.

Using Negative Calorie Foods

If you find that you are hungry between meals, eating negative calorie foods can help you to control your caloric intake.

Foods like carrots, celery and other vegetables and fruits that are not considered starches can be used to fill in points in your day when you experience break through hunger.

ACTION PLAN

Chia seeds can be cooked or sprinkled raw over your food. If you are looking to add a little bit of crunch or texture to your dish, then serving them as a toasted garnish on the top of your dish can add a lot of depth.

Everyday Habit #60

Negative Calorie Foods Cheat Sheet

Negative calorie foods are a great way to ensure that you lose weight and we have mentioned them multiple times in this book. However, without knowing what negative calorie foods really are, it doesn't do you much good. So, we created a cheat sheet for you that will help you to develop a better diet. This cheat sheet consists of negative calorie fruits, vegetables and spices that will help you to create the perfect meal plan for you and your family, while still making sure that your meals taste great and fill you up.

Mixing in negative calorie fruits and vegetables will provide you with more food without adding extra calories to your meal.

What is a Negative Calorie Food?

Negative calorie foods do contain calories; so, don't let the name fool you. However, because of the makeup of these foods, the density of the foods and the energy it takes to process and digest the food, your body burns more calories breaking them down than they actually contain.

Negative Calorie Fruits

Negative calorie fruits are extremely tasty. You can eat pretty much as much as you want without gaining weight. This makes them the perfect snack between meals, or the addition to a high calorie side dish. These fruits should be eaten in their raw form to be considered negative calorie. The fruit should not be packed in syrup or processed in any way.

- Apples
- Blueberries
- Cantaloupe
- Cranberries
- Grapefruits
- Honeydew melon
- Lemons
- Limes
- Mangoes
- Oranges
- Papaya
- Peaches
- Pineapple
- Raspberries
- Strawberries
- Tangerines
- Watermelon

Negative Calorie Vegetables

It is important to note that in order to be considered negative calorie vegetables, these veggies must be eaten in their raw form or steamed. They should not be microwaved, or have any additive other than negative calorie seasonings added to them.

- Asparagus
- Bean Sprouts
- Beets
- Broccoli

- Cabbage
- Carrots
- Cauliflower
- Celery
- Chicory
- Radicchio
- Cucumbers
- Endives
- Green beans
- Jicama
- Kale
- Leeks
- Lettuce
- Radishes
- Spinach
- Squash
- Tomatoes
- Turnips
- Zucchini

Negative Calorie Herbs and Spices

Herbs and spices are a great way to add flavor to your food.

The herbs and spices that are listed here are considered negative calorie in their fresh and dried forms.

- Anise
- Cayenne
- Chili peppers
- Cinnamon
- Cloves
- Coriander
- Cilantro

- Cumin
- Dill
- Fennel seeds
- Flax seeds
- Garden cress
- Garlic
- Ginger
- Parsley
- Onion
- Mustard seeds
- Watercress

Starchy Vegetables that You Should Limit

There are certain vegetables that fall into the starch/carbohydrate category that are still eaten as a vegetable, and even worse, next to another starch.

These specific vegetables should serve as the starch/carbohydrate if they are on your plate as you should never eat a double carbohydrate at any meal.

- Baked beans
- Corn
- Green Peas
- Plantains
- Potatoes
- Squash
- Sweet potato family

Everyday Habit #61

Know Your Carbohydrates

Since a large majority of your calories should come from your carbohydrate intake, we have decided that it would be valuable for you to have a resource to refer to when it comes to your carbohydrates and starch sources.

Whole Grains

Breads	
Item	**Serving**
Whole Wheat Bagel	1 ounce or ¼ of a bagel
Whole Wheat Crackers	2 to 5 crackers
Whole Wheat English Muffins	1 cup
Whole Wheat Hamburger Buns	½ muffin
Whole Wheat Bread	½ bun
Melba Toasts	4 slices
Whole Wheat Pita (6-inch diameter)	½ pita
Pumpernickel Bread	1 Slice
Whole Wheat Rice Cake	2 rice cakes
Whole Wheat Roll	1 roll
Rye Bread	1 slice
Whole Wheat Tortilla (6-inch diameter)	1 tortilla
Grains	
Item	**Serving**

Barley	½ cup
Bran Cereal	½ cup
Brown Rice	½ cup
Buckwheat	½ cup
Bulgur	½ cup
Whole Wheat Cereal	½ cup
Whole Wheat Couscous	½ cup
Low Fat Granola	½ cup
Grape Nuts	½ cup
Kasha	½ cup
Whole Wheat Macaroni	½ cup
Millet	½ cup
Muesli	½ cup
Oats	½ cup
Whole Wheat Pasta	½ cup
Quinoa	½ cup
Shredded Wheat	½ cup
Wheat Germ	3 tbsp

Starchy Vegetables

Baked Beans	½ cup
Corn	½ cup
Corn on the Cob	½ cup
Mixed Vegetables with Corn, Peas or Pasta	½ cup
Boiled Potatoes	½ cup
Baked potato (with skin)	½ cup
Mashed Potatoes	½ cup
Plain yams or sweet potatoes	½ cup

Legumes

Beans and Peas	½ cup
Lima Beans	½ cup
Lentils	½ cup
Miso Paste	3 Tbsp

Misc. Grains and Starches

Animal Crackers	8 crackers
White Bagel	¼ bagel
White Bread	1 slice
Bread Sticks, 4" x 1/2"	4 sticks
Cornmeal	3 tbsp
English Muffin	½ muffin
Graham Crackers, 2 ½" square	3 crackers
Grits	½ cup
Hot Dog Bun	½ bun
Matzoh	¾ ounce
Naan, 8"x 2"	¼
Oyster Crackers	20 crackers
Pancakes, 4" across, ¼" thick	1 pancake
Pasta	½ cup cooked
Popcorn (Air popped)	3 cups
Pretzels	¾ ounce
Raisin Bread (no frosting)	1 slice
Rice Cakes	2 rice cakes
White rice	½ cup cooked
Saltine Crackers	6 crackers
Corn Tortillas (6" diameter)	1 tortilla
Flour Tortilla's (6" diameter)	1 tortilla

Starchy Foods Prepared with Fat Products

Crackers, round buttered style	6 crackers

Croutons (unseasoned)	1 cup
French Fries	1 cup
Granola	¼ cup
Peanut Butter or Cheese Filled Sandwich Crackers	3 crackers
Chowmein noodles	1/3 cup
Potato Chips	9 to 12 chips
Tortilla Chips	9 to 12 chips
Hummus	1/3 cup
Microwaved Popcorn	3 cups
Cooked Stuffing	1/3 cup
Whole Wheat Crackers with Added Fat	4 to 7 crackers
Biscuits 2 ½" across	1 biscuit
Corn Bread 2" cube	1 cube
Waffle 4" across	1 waffle
Muffin, 5 ounces	1/5 of a muffin or one ounce
Taco Shell, 5 Across	2 taco shells (not including fillings)

As you can see, it is not necessary to avoid foods that are considered unhealthy. However, it is important to only consume these items in moderation. These foods can be a great addition to your diet as long as you follow the recommended serving sizes and you do not over indulge in these foods.

Bonus Tips

As you know, your weight and the way you feel directly translate into the way you perceive yourself, or your self-esteem. Not only does it influence the way you feel about yourself, but it can also influence the way you feel about the world around you. By making good food choices that are healthy and have a positive impact on your weight and the chemicals that your brain releases, you can change the way you feel about yourself and the way you look at the world around you. Exercise can also have a huge impact on how you feel and the way you perceive yourself.

Your Habits Translate to Your Self-Esteem

Not only can your habits translate into the way you physically feel, it can also have a positive or negative effect on your self-esteem, or the way you feel about yourself. If you have had low self-esteem for a long time, or you have tried diet after diet and failed taking the risk of making positive changes in your life can seem a bit intimidating.

Making Positive Changes

By making positive changes in your life, even if they are one at a time, you get the satisfaction of taking control of your life as a whole and taking control of your health. Succeeding in making a positive change and developing a positive habit you can increase your self-esteem and empower yourself to make other changes. This is why we have presented positive changes that you can make in your life one at a time.

Do A Little at A Time

By changing your life in small increments, you make overall success more possible. As you create a habit and experience how much better you feel in general, you will become more excited about the future and how each change you make will help you feel better and better. If your health, or your current eating habits, are difficult to overcome, take tiny steps toward your overall goal. Even the steps we have outlined in this book can be broken down into smaller steps that will lead to your overall goal. If you have allowed your stamina to diminish to the point where all you can offer is three minutes of exercise, make those three minutes count.

Three minutes of getting up and moving is better than not trying at all. Not ready to call it "exercising" yet? You don't have to! Simply getting up and cleaning your house can burn a lot of calories and give you proof of your progress, proof that you can see and feel at the same time.

Keep a Journal

By keeping a journal that outlines your physical stamina and the way you feel on a daily basis can help you to make positive changes in your life. When you hit a rough patch, you can look at your journal and the changes you have made so far. You can see what you have overcome and how much your life has changed since you began instating changes. Seeing your struggles and your triumphs can give you the motivation you need to get through rough spots in changing your diet, increasing your exercise and developing a healthier life.

Even though we offer these tips, we cannot promise that any change in your life will be easy. If you want to have more energy, live a better life, feel better about yourself, lose weight and live longer, you have to have the drive and motivation to make these changes.

Analyzing Our Recommendations

Since everyone is different, it is important for you to analyze all of our recommendations and determine which changes will benefit your life, which changes you should start with, and which changes will provide you the motivation to carry through with the rest. Choose a change that will be easy for you first, so that you can begin to accept change and see it in a positive way.

In your journal, plan your changes in the order you think will benefit your life so that you know what to look forward to, and you can mentally and emotionally prepare yourself for each change before you reach your start date. Take your time as you go through these steps and make sure that you give yourself time to develop a true habit out of each step before moving on to the next goal.

Talk to Your Doctor

Just like any other serious change in your life, you should talk to your doctor about your plans and ask if there are any specific concerns they have because of any current health conditions you have, or any health conditions you are predisposed to developing. Ask for your doctor's advice for your specific situation before beginning any serious life change, especially if it involves adding a supplement, or exercise to your current regimen. If you have current health conditions, your doctor may advise you against trying one of our suggestions, or they may instruct you to modify the suggestion in various ways until your health improves.

Consulting a Nutritionist

If you have diabetes, or you have certain food intolerances, you may want to consult a dietician or nutritionist. They can help you modify some of our recommendations to suit your current dietary needs or intolerances.

Don't Stop Here!

There are hundreds of other ways that you can improve your life and the way you feel. The recommendations that we have presented in this book are a great starting point for developing better overall health and can be expanded upon very easily, especially once you have reached the goals here. Expanding upon your nutritional and fitness goals will help you to feel better and develop better health than you could ever imagine. These recommendations are for those who are ready to start taking control of their weight, the way they feel, and start the journey to physical fitness and better self-esteem.

Take Your Time

When it comes to weight loss and getting yourself back in shape, there is no reason to rush. Take your time and lose weight in effective, proven ways that are considered safe in general, and check with your doctor to make sure that they are safe for you. Will you drop 100 pounds in a month? No! Do not expect to lose weight fast and if you begin losing weight too fast, you should consult your doctor. With the proper diet and exercise, you can safely lose three pounds per week of fat. However, you may see pretty quick results at the beginning from initial water weight, especially if your doctor, nutritionist, or dietician recommends a flush to begin your diet changes.

A flush will help to rid your body of toxins and excess water weight. A water weight flush can help you to lose nine pounds in the initial week that you begin your diet change. However, you should only do this if your doctor or dietician approves. Once the water weight has been removed, you will be able to focus on burning fat instead of fighting with water weight. For many people, this is a positive way to start your new life and your approach to making the changes in your life because it shows you that what goes on with your body is completely under your control.

Will These Changes Affect Your Entire Family?

If the changes you are making will affect your entire family, it is recommended that you consult with each family member's physician. Each person should have a complete physical and be tested for allergies that could potentially stand in their way. You should also review the plan change with each person's physician to ensure that they are healthy enough for the proposed physical activity, as well as the diet changes that will take place.

Consult with a dietician to determine the best way to make these changes with your children. Once a child is used to eating a certain diet, it may be difficult to get them to accept the change. Dieticians who specialize in treating children know tips and tricks to get children to eat foods that they have not been previously introduced to.

Allow Your Kids to Help Prepare Meals

By allowing your children to help prepare meals, you are allowing them to have some control over what they are eating, and empower them to try new things. This is especially true if your children are extremely hesitant to try new foods.

Nothing is truly "Off Limits"

Even though certain foods are healthier for you than others that do not provide the same health benefits. However, you must learn to enjoy these foods only in moderation, and you must be able to enjoy the foods in small quantities. If you do choose to indulge in foods that are less than healthy, you must ensure that you take into account these calories when determining your daily calorie intake.

Eating Healthy Does Not Mean Depriving Yourself

Eating healthy does not mean that you have to deprive yourself of the delicious treats in life. It simply means that you must retrain your body to acknowledge them as treats instead of as a staple item in your diet. The majority of your calories will need to come from healthy sources, however on rare occasion, some of your calories can come from a treat, as long as it is in moderation.

Extra Bonus Advice!

The secret to health and happiness is cultivating good habits. These habits work as the foundation upon which the rest of your life is built. If your habits are unhealthy, your foundation is weak and at risk of falling apart. Healthy habits that nurture your body and mind provide a strong foundation that will make everything else in your life run more smoothly.

A healthy diet and plenty of exercise are the cornerstones of this foundation but there are other healthy habits that you probably never even thought to include. This book is meant to provide you with a look into 12 of those unique habits that are all too easy to overlook but still essential to a healthy, happy life. Each of the following chapters focuses on a specific habit. You'll learn what the habit is, how it affects your health and wellbeing, and get specific steps and strategies for incorporating the habit into your own routine.

Remember: the key to making long-term, sustainable lifestyle changes (like adopting new habits) is to pace yourself. Don't try to start doing all 12 of these habits at once. You might succeed for the first couple of days but you'll soon get frustrated and fall back into your old habits. You're setting yourself up for disappointment if you try to tackle them all at the same time. So, to avoid disappointment and failure, work on cultivating one habit at a time. Slowly add in new habits at a pace that works for you. I recommend adding one habit each week. As you add in a new habit, remember to continue working on the habits you have already added.

By slowly adding new habits one week at a time, you give yourself the time to get used to the small, gradual changes that you are making to your lifestyle. The transition to a new, healthier lifestyle will be so smooth, you will hardly realize that anything has changed—except for the fact that you'll feel healthier, more energetic, less stressed out, and just generally happier with your body and your life!

The habits you'll learn about in this book include simple changes like taking off your shoes when you come in the house as well as bigger changes like learning to manage and release your anger in healthy ways. Each of these habits will help you get healthier (physically and emotionally) which will make losing weight easier and taking on bigger habit changes (like diet changes or adding exercise routines) much easier to handle. So keep reading and get ready to make some changes to your lifestyle so that you can feel healthier and happier in your new life!

Everyday Habit #62

Punch Something!

That's right. This habit is to punch something. Now, I'm not trying to advocate violence or get you arrested (I promise!). But studies have shown that letting out your anger and frustration through physical activity is essential for your health. So, punch a punching bag or punch a pillow (or anything else that you can punch without risking jail time).

Bottling up your anger and frustration and trying to keep calm can actually cause serious damage to your physical health (not to mention your emotional health). Studies show that holding in your rage leads to dangerously high blood pressure, poor concentration, lack of focus, and trouble sleeping. That last one (sleeping troubles) leads to a host of other health problems you don't want to deal with.

Before you can really understand *why* you need to let that anger out (in safe, non-deadly ways), you have to understand *how* your body is affected by anger.

Here's the chain reaction that happens in your body when you feel anger:

First, your nervous system kicks into high gear. The nervous system is what sends messages from your brain to the rest of your body. The angry messages coming from your brain travel through your nervous system and reach every part of your body. When these messages reach your heart, it results in a faster heart rate. This increased heart rate leads to higher blood pressure and more blood being delivered to your muscles. These messages also tell your body to start producing adrenalin, which stops your body from producing insulin at the same time that it boosts glucose levels in your blood. Lower insulin and high glucose levels are what give you that boost of energy that is associated with adrenalin.

All of this is happening because your body is assuming that the anger is the result of a physical threat. It is getting itself ready for quick action. That is, it's getting ready for either a fight or flight response (both of which need a lot of extra energy). So, when you try to push down the anger instead of release it, you are physically bottling up all that extra energy.

The more you get angry and the more you try to bottle it up, the more stress you are putting on your body by filling it up with excess energy that never gets released. This leads to consistently high blood pressure (even when you are not angry), digestive problems, weakened immune system, and other weakened systems because the constant pressure and stress you are putting on your physical body by trying to contain your emotional responses wears it down. By releasing that anger in healthy ways, you are using up that excess energy. You are giving your body the feeling that it has done something productive to respond to the threat. Even if your anger is not caused by someone or something that is an actual threat to your health or wellbeing, your body will assume this is what's happening and will want to do what it can to fight or flee the situation.

Going through the motions of fighting (or fleeing) will send your body the signal that the problem has been dealt with and it can return to normal. That way, you are not putting excessive stress on your body or forcing it to remain under constant pressure. So, make it a habit to release your anger in healthy and safe ways so that your body can rest easily, knowing that it is safe to relax and restore itself to a normal, healthy state.

ACTION PLAN

If you aren't really sure how to begin releasing your anger in positive ways or are still convinced that punching your boss in the face is a "healthy" expression of your frustration, then try out these steps and strategies for making anger release a part of your regular routine.

First of all, try to estimate how severe your anger problems are. Answer the following questions about your own anger:

1. About how many times per week (on average) do you get angry?
2. Think about the last thing that made you angry. Does the same intensity of anger come back when you think about it?
3. Have people close to you said that you have a temper?
4. Do you feel that you are quick to anger?

If you find that you are getting angry on a daily basis or you answered yes to questions 2, 3, or 4, then you might be in need of anger management therapy. These questions cannot provide a diagnosis but they may offer a sign that you are having troubles controlling your anger or releasing it in effective ways. Even if you don't have a temper or any specific issues with anger management, you could still benefit from releasing your rage when it does happen. Even the most calm and peaceful people can be driven to rage given the right (or, more likely, the wrong) circumstances.

Try these steps for releasing your frustrations before they cause excessive strain on your body or long-term damage to your health:

Step 1: Channel your anger.

If you are in the habit of repressing your anger and keeping it bottled up, you need to start by working through old anger. Think of it like going on a detox diet. In order to restore your body, you'll have to pull out all the toxins (in this case, anger) that have been building up in your body and flush them all out.

Think about the last time you were angry. Recall every detail of the situation and the way that you felt at the time. Except this time, instead of trying to hold that anger in, allow yourself to feel it. Pay attention to the physical changes in your body as this old anger starts to take effect. Feel your breathing get faster. Feel your heart starting to race. Feel your cheeks start to flush with heat from the increased blood pressure.

Step 2: Write it down.

Describe the situation that made you angry. Describe the way you felt. Try to explain the connections between these two things. Explain in detail what it was about this situation that made you so angry. Explain why it was that you tried to push the anger down instead of let it out. This process of writing is the first step in releasing the anger that you have just reawakened in yourself. It's allowing you to wake it up even more at the same time that you are starting to give it a small amount of release.

Step 3: Pour it out.

The act of writing it down is cathartic in itself but it is still not enough to release the pent-up physical energy coursing through your body. To let out this physical part of your anger, you need to do something physical. The title of this chapter recommends punching something but you can also do any other physical activity that helps you feel that release.

Try lifting weights, going for a run, rock climbing, or any other physical activity that really works your muscle. Push yourself when you do this activity. Your body is full of energy and ready to go into high gear. It doesn't want to take a peaceful walk or go fishing. It wants to charge at full speed and smash things. Give your body this satisfaction by doing a workout that pushes you to your limits. Don't strain yourself or push *beyond* your limits (you could also cause damage this way) but do allow your body to reach maximum capacity.

Everyday Habit #63

This Habit Will Surprise You!

After getting pumped about releasing your anger, you might be a little shocked to learn that the next habit you should be working on is something as mundane sounding as cleaning. But it's true. In order to improve your health, you should get in the habit of cleaning your home every day. That doesn't mean doing a total overhaul every day. In fact, if you get into this habit, the cleaning will only get easier and easier. Your home will be consistently clean so you'll only have to do a few things here and there each day to maintain the standard. You might be thinking: ok, sure, it'll get easier when the house is clean but how on earth could cleaning every day affect my health? Well, there are a few different reasons for that. Some are physical and some are psychological. Taken altogether, this habit will improve your physical health *and* your overall quality of life at the same time.

Let's start with the physical side. Cleaning is a physical activity, which means it burns calories. Granted, it's definitely not burning as many calories as a run or a 30-minute weight lifting session. But it's still going to make a dent in your total number of calories burned—especially if you do cleaning that gets your heart pumping faster. In addition to being a good way to get your body moving (which comes with its own long list of health benefits), it's also better for your health in other ways. Cleaning your home isn't just about organizing things and putting everything where it goes. It also means using soap and water and scrubbing down the surfaces. It means vacuuming all the dirt and organisms living in your carpets. It means wiping away the dust that would otherwise float through the air and get inhaled by you into your lungs. Overall, a clean home is a home that has significantly less bacteria, germs, and allergens. When you keep your home consistently tidy, you're helping cut down on your risk of getting sick or developing an allergy.

Enough of the physical benefits, what about the psychological benefits? Recent studies have found that people tend to behave more nicely and feel more generous if they are in a clean smelling room. This means you will feel more positive and optimistic about the world in general if you just keep your home clean. There are countless studies that show what a key role the environment you are in plays in terms of psychological health. For example, imagine you are going to therapy to work through some emotional issues you have.

Would you prefer to get that therapy in a cluttered, dusty basement with old, moldy food containers lying around or would you want to get therapy in a clean, spacious, and organized room? When you are surrounded by disorder, unpleasant smells, and hazardous materials (like broken glass or molding foods), your stress levels go up and you have a hard time concentrating on any task. Keeping your physical space clean, organized, and pleasant will translate to feeling as if your entire life is more organized and under control. You will have an easier time focusing on the task at hand and you will find it more relaxing to be at home in general.

ACTION PLAN

There's no excuse not to clean your house every day. If you have a busy schedule or 5 messy kids or just plain don't feel like it, there's still a way to make sure you get your daily cleaning accomplished. Use these strategies to help you make sure you keep your home clean:

Take a weekend to do a deep clean.

If you aren't already in the habit of cleaning on a daily basis, you've probably let a few chores go neglected. Use a weekend or a day off to give your house a complete, thorough wash down. Clean every nook and cranny—even the ones where you usually try to hide messes! Throw out things you don't need and eliminate clutter. Reorganize your closet and invest in drawers, shelves, and other methods of storage to help you keep your stuff organized. Transform your home into a clean, organized, and relaxing space.

Don't let messes build up.

After you cook, clean the dishes (or at least load them into the dishwasher). The same goes for after you finish eating. When you change out of work clothes in the evening, put them into the laundry basket instead of on the floor or a chair. Scrub the toilet as soon as you notice it's dirty (this will prevent tough stains). When you see a dirty spot on the fridge or on a table, clean it right then and there. Get in the habit of cleaning things as soon as you notice they need a cleaning.

Make time in your schedule.

If you are busy and have a tight schedule, try to squeeze 15 to 20 minutes here and there to take care of your home. In many cases, you can multitask. Start a load of laundry and then go load the dishwasher and vacuum while both machines are doing their thing.

You'll be surprised how much you can get done in 20 minutes if you focus on cleaning and find optimal ways to multitask. Even 20 minutes of cleaning each day will add up and help keep your home tidy. By cleaning a little bit each day, you can avoid spending your days off catching up on housework.

Learn to Prioritize.

This one applies especially to those of you who have kids. Kids can be like tornadoes of mess in an otherwise clean home. As a parent, you probably feel like any attempt to clean is futile. It's true, with kids, your home just isn't going to be as clean as it could be. So, you're going to have to learn to prioritize. Focus on taking care of messes that could turn into biohazards: food spills, mud tracked through the house, toilet accidents, and so on. If you don't clean these immediately, they become breeding grounds for bacteria, germs, and other things you don't want in your home. You'll have to learn to live with some scattered toys and clothes strewn about but at least you'll be able to find time for the immediate health risks.

Teach good habits.

This is another one for the parents out there. Start getting your children involved in the housework at an early age. When they are still toddlers, you can start them on simple tasks. At such a young age, they probably won't actually be much help but you will be teaching good habits that will make it much easier for you to get them to help with the chores when they get older. This way, your kids will eventually become a source of help in keeping the home clean rather than an adorable little harbinger of destruction.

Enjoying this book?

Check out my other best sellers!

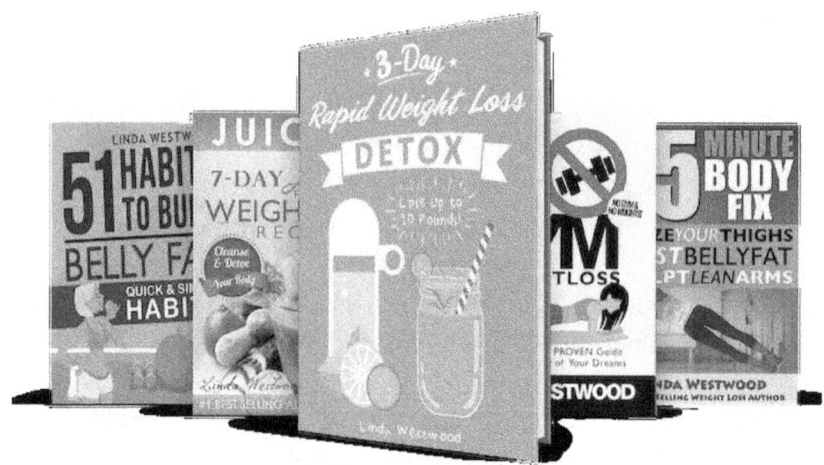

Get your next book on sale here:

TopFitnessAdvice.com/go/books

Everyday Habit #64

Walk Around Barefoot (At Home)

After working on the habit from the previous chapter, your home will be nice and clean. So, take off your shoes and enjoy your newly cleaned home. Doing so will actually help keep your home even cleaner. The bottoms of your shoes get tracked through all manner of grime and gunk and stuff you don't really want to deal with—which is why you wear shoes in the first place, so you don't have to step on that stuff in your bare feet.

If you wear your shoes inside the house, you are tracking all those germs and toxic chemicals from outside all through your house. These harmful toxins can cause all sorts of problems from dementia and Alzheimer's disease to childhood leukemia and obesity. That is to say: these toxins can ruin your quality of life from childhood through to old age. So, take your shoes off at the door and leave them there. You can wear socks, slippers, or just go bare foot—whichever feels more comfortable to you. Just do not wear shoes in the house. There's no reason to do it anyway. Shoes are made with the purpose of protecting your feet when you go outside. When you're at home, there's not any risk of stepping on broken glass or dog poop or any of the other things you need to avoid outside.

There are additional benefits to freeing your feet at home. First of all, it allows them to breathe. Yes, your feet need to breathe. Sweat, bacteria, and microbes build up in your shoes all day long and if you don't allow your feet to escape for a while, you could end up with athlete's foot, other fungal infections, or even just a serious case of unbearably stinky feet. It may also be good for your posture. In shoes (especially poorly fitting, uncomfortable shoes), your feet are bent into strange positions that can put pressure on the wrong parts of your feet. When you are barefoot, your foot is able to be in its natural position so that it can distribute the pressure of your weight evenly and comfortably.

ACTION PLAN

Your action plan here is going to be pretty simple: take off your shoes when you get home. Leave them off until you need to go outside again. To avoid forgetting to do this, place a shelf or mat next to the door that will act as your designated shoe area. Put a pair of shoes that you rarely wear on the shelf or mat so that you are immediately reminded of what it's there for.

Each time you get home, take your shoes off and put them on the shelf or mat (just as you put your keys on a hook or in a bowl). This will easily become a habit, as you'll quickly realize what a stress relief it is to be able to shut the front door and take your shoes off. It's a great way to send yourself the message "finally, I'm home and I'm here to stay." If you are really having trouble remembering to do it, set a reminder on your phone that goes off at the time that you normally walk in the front door.

Everyday Habit #65

Take More Naps!

Yes, you read that right. Take more naps! Sleep is essential and keeping your mind well rested is the key to productivity. Multiple studies have shown that people who work less and rest more actually tend to be *more* productive than people who work overtime and are chronically sleep deprived. This might sound counterintuitive but it makes sense when you look at the physical processes behind it. People who don't give their body the rest it needs are working in a constant state of stress. Their bodies are getting worn down more and more from the consistent high stress levels and the lack of rest is preventing them from repairing the damage caused by that stress. To add to this dangerous cycle, the increased stress makes it even more difficult to fall asleep or get any kind of quality rest (which means it becomes even more difficult for the body to take time to repair itself).

On the other hand, people who do take naps may work less total hours in a day but during the hours they are working, they are even more productive than those who don't take naps. This is because rest is not just about turning off your brain. It's about giving your brain the time it needs to patch up any damages and strengthen neural connections. Even as you are sleeping, your brain is still very much active and working to restore you to optimal health and productivity. Nap takers have improved cognitive skills (including focus, alertness, memory, and problem-solving skills). They also have lower blood pressure, lower stress, and an almost 40% lower risk for heart attack. This means that taking naps can make you a happier, less stressed out person overall *and* a more productive worker at the same time!

ACTION PLAN

You might find it hard to fit naps into a busy schedule but keep in mind that napping is going to make you more productive so don't think of it so much as taking a break from work as making naps a key *part* of work. Think of it as rebooting your brain just as you would reboot a computer if it started to run too slowly. The ideal length of a power nap is between 10 and 20 minutes. This allows your body and mind to achieve a state of restfulness without going into deep sleep (which could result in some grogginess after waking up).

So, aim to keep your naps within the 10 to 20 minutes range during the day in order to avoid messing with your sleep schedule at night. The ideal time to schedule your nap is between 1pm and 3pm. This is in line with your biological clock. We naturally tend to lose a little momentum by this time of day (assuming a wake-up time of between 5am and 8am) so it's the perfect time to let your brain reboot. This time frame is also far enough away from your regular sleeping time that you won't cause any trouble with trying to keep your normal sleep schedule.

In terms of falling asleep for your nap:

- **Don't stress about actually falling asleep:** when you first start to nap, you might not actually fall asleep. Just focus on resting your mind and body and enjoying the calm before you dive back into the storm.

- **Find a dark, calm place:** turn off your light and shut your office door or go sit in your car and recline the seat all the way back. You want darkness (or at least low light) and calm (but not necessarily quiet) so that your mind doesn't get distracted.

- **Use white noise:** during the day, the world can be a very noisy place. Your mind might be trying to focus on all the different sounds. Give it some white noise that can help drown out the noises of the day and give your mind a single point of focus. This can be the sound of a fan or a soundtrack of ocean waves. It can even be music so long as it is instrumental and doesn't have lyrics. If you use music, it should also be relatively slow or calming rather than upbeat or fast paced. Classical music can be great for this.

If you are worried that your boss or coworkers might disapprove of your new napping habit, try explaining your logic. Send them some informative links or point them to this book so that they can see how napping can actually improve workplace productivity. Who knows, maybe you'll even inspire your boss to institute an official afternoon naptime!

Everyday Habit #66

Use A Neti Pot

The fifth habit you should develop looks pretty strange but it is extremely beneficial to your health. If you've never heard of a neti pot, it's a pretty simple device. It's shaped somewhat like a small watering pot and it's used to pour salt water up one nasal canal and out the other. Why would you ever pour water up your nose on purpose, you may ask? It's a method of nasal irrigation. It clears out mucus build-up and opens up your sinuses so that you can breathe better and avoid infection.

If you are already suffering from a stuffy nose, the neti pot will help you recover more quickly. If you are still breathing normally, it can help prevent infections before they start. The neti pot is much more effective and much less harmful than blowing your nose. When you blow your nose, you are placing a lot of pressure on your sinuses. You have also probably noticed the pain and chaffing of repeatedly blowing and wiping your nose. By using a neti pot, you can clear out your sinuses and nasal passages quickly and painlessly without leaving your nose red and chaffed. You also clear much more out with the neti pot than you would just by blowing your nose.

Using the neti pot regularly (although not daily) is a great way to boost your overall health. It will help keep infectious bacteria or irritating allergens to a minimum and help you breathe more easily in the long term. Use it about 3 times per week when you are healthy and daily when you are congested.

ACTION PLAN

Using a neti pot is simple but there are a few things you need to keep in mind. First, we'll go over the basic process then we'll talk about how to avoid some of the most common mistakes people make when using it.

1. Pour 2 cups of water into a pot.
2. Add 1 teaspoon of salt.
3. Bring the pot to a boil.
4. Let it cool to room temperature.
5. Pour this into your neti pot.
6. Insert the tip of the neti pot into one nostril.
7. Lean your head sideways over a sink.
8. Lift the neti pot up (while making sure that the tip stays in your nose) until you feel the salt water solution pouring into your nostril.
9. It will begin to pour out of the other nostril into the sink.
10. Repeat this process but pouring the water into the opposite nostril this time.

That's the basic process. Now, here's what you need to keep in mind:

First of all, when the salt-water solution pours out of the opposite nostril, it's going to be carrying a lot of gunk with it. It will look gross. But it's better to have that gunk in the sink than in your nose, right?

Secondly, the salt you add should be ground sea salt or kosher salt. Make sure to check that there are no other additives in the salt. In common table salt, manufacturers tend to add ingredients that prevent it from clumping up. This is fine for the salt but less fine for your nose.

Next, always boil the water. Unless you are using pure, distilled water, you always want to boil the water to make sure it is sanitized. If you pour water that's not sanitized into your nose, you'll cause a lot more harm than good. To be on the safe side, always boil the water. Boiling also helps to dissolve the salt more quickly so you don't have painful grains of salt inside your nose. Always thoroughly wash your neti pot after each use, dry it completely, and store it in a dry, safe place. With all that in mind, as weird as it might sound, it's really not uncomfortable and it's great for your health.

Everyday Habit #67

Clean Cash

Money is dirty. I don't mean the "illegal" kind of dirty. I mean the filthy, germ-riddled kind of dirty. It's been passed through so many hands and stuck in so many unclean places that it is literally (and I mean scientifically proven to be) as dirty as a public toilet. You don't have to give up money and live as a hermit in the woods. Just pay with your card when you can and wash your hands if you handle money. You don't have to use any special, extra powerful cleanser. Warm soap and water will do the trick. Treat handling money the same way you treat using a public toilet.

Washing your hands regularly just makes sense in general. The world is filled with bacteria and germs. Sure, lots of them are harmless and some are even beneficial but there are definitely plenty of dangerous, mean bacteria out there that you don't want living on your hands and spreading to your mouth, nose, or eyes. You can't avoid coming into contact with these dangerous germs unless you decide to cut off all contact with the outside world and live in a sealed bubble. So, there's no reason to panic and try to avoid all contact. Just make sure to wash your hands regularly and avoid touching your eyes, mouth, nose, or ears after handling money or using a public toilet (at least until you have washed your hands).

ACTION PLAN

To make sure that hand washing is effective, use soap and warm water. Massage the soap into your hands and wrists for at least 30 seconds before rinsing it off in warm water again. You don't need to use antibacterial soaps. These are not any more effective than regular soap and can actually cause harm in the long run. If you look at a bottle of antibacterial soap, you'll see that it never claims to be 100% effective. It always says something like "99.99%", and in most situations in life that kind of statistic sounds like a sure thing—it's basically 100%, right?

In the case of bacteria, the opposite is true. That 0.01% of bacteria that survive the antibacterial chemical in the soap will reproduce themselves on your hands, producing even more of the kind of bacteria that are resistant to that soap. This means that each time you use an antibacterial soap (or hand sanitizer), it becomes less effective than it was before. At the same time, it breeds even more resistant, stronger bacteria than before. This will put you at an even higher risk than you were before. So, avoid antibacterial soaps (and hand sanitizers). Instead, just use normal soap and warm water. By massaging the soap in for at least 30 seconds and rinsing thoroughly, you will successfully wash away the bacteria.

Everyday Habit #68

Shut the Lid!

This one is deceptively simple: shut the lid of the toilet before you flush. As easy as it sounds, it is really easy to forget to do this but it's worth taping up a huge sign on your bathroom door to make sure everyone in the house remembers. Dr. Charles Gerba, a microbiologist working at the University of Arizona, explains that the force of flushing the toilet sends water particles (polluted with waste debris) up into the air. These particles can float around for a few hours before finally settling on all surfaces of the bathroom and even your toothbrush.

While these particles are harmless in most cases, on rare occasions, they can carry E Coli and other harmful bacteria that you don't want living on your toothbrush, make up, or any other bathroom products. In reality, you probably don't find the idea of brushing your teeth with harmless fecal-based bacteria all that appealing either. Even if it's not harmful, it's still pretty gross. To avoid coating everything in your bathroom in a fine layer of waste particles, shut the lid *before* you flush the toilet. Make it a habit to keep the lid closed any time the toilet is not in use. This way, waste particles and bacteria stay safely trapped in the toilet and far away from your toothbrush or shower sponge. You can consider this part of your habit of cleaning every day. This habit will help make sure that you maintain a high level of sanitation and cleanliness in your bathroom.

The bathroom is an especially important area of the house to keep clean because it's where you go to eliminate waste and wash off germs and bacteria—which means that your toilet, sink, shower and other bathroom areas quickly become full of those same germs and bacteria that you cleaned off of yourself. Keep the bathroom as clean as possible to avoid letting those bacteria multiply and find their way back onto your skin or worse, into your mouth, ears, eyes, or nose where they can cause serious infection.

ACTION PLAN

Before this becomes a fully-fledged habit, it is going to be hard to remember to do this (and even harder to get the other members of your household on track with it, too). Here are some tips to help you remember to do it and help get everyone else in the habit as well:

Put up a sign.

Post a simple sign with something like "Close the lid before you flush" in the bathroom. Make sure it is somewhere that you see while sitting on the toilet (or above the toilet so that you see it when you go to flush). Use colors that attract attention so that you don't ignore it. Red has been shown to attract the most attention (which is why it's so often used in warning signs). Also use highly contrasting colors so that the sign really stands out (like bright red on a white background). This may not be the most beautiful decoration but you only need to keep it up for a few weeks. Once everyone is in the habit of closing the lid, you can take it down.

Explain the logic.

Tell the other members of your household why it's so important to close the lid before flushing. They will probably be equally disgusted by the thought of having fecal bacteria on their stuff as well. If they understand why they're doing it, they'll be more likely to put the effort into making it a habit.

Make a trigger.

One trick to making any habit stick is to develop a trigger that reminds you to do it. For example, people trying to wake up earlier will get up in exactly the same way each morning. This ritual of waking up the same way works as a trigger to get your mind in the right gear. To get in the habit of closing the lid, set up a new toilet ritual.

For example, when you get into the bathroom and see that the lid is open, try closing it and then opening it again. Ideally, when the habit is in place, you will have to open the lid each time you use the toilet (because it should be closed whenever it's not in use). Shutting and opening the lid before you use the toilet will trigger your memory to close it before flushing.

Be in the moment.

It's easy to use the toilet without paying so much attention to what you are doing. You use the toilet every single day (usually multiple times per day) so it becomes a sort of unconscious routine. Since shutting the lid is not yet part of that unconscious routine, you need to work on being conscious of everything you are doing so that your mind doesn't wander off, leaving your body to go through the routine motions.

Pay attention to everything from closing the door and sitting down to counting how many squares of toilet paper you pull off the roll. You can explicitly tell yourself what you are doing to help you stay present and in the moment. For example, when shutting the door, say, "I am shutting the door." It might feel silly or awkward but again, you only have to do this while you are trying to develop the habit. Once it becomes part of your regular routine, you'll be able to shut the lid without having to consciously think about it.

Everyday Habit #69

Natural Migraine Destroyer

This habit might sound a little out there but there are actually scientific studies to back it up. If you have a migraine, smell an apple to help alleviate the pain. In a recent study done at Chicago's Smell & Taste Treatment and Research Foundation, researchers found that the scent of a green apple reduced the intensity of migraine pain. This may be less to do with any specific chemical compounds in the odor and more to do with the relaxation power of pleasant scents. This is the theory behind the general practice of aromatherapy for treating migraines and headaches. The pleasant scent triggers the pleasure receptors in your brain.

These pleasure receptors work to decrease the pain response in your body, lower your stress levels, and send soothing signals throughout your nervous system. That means that, in addition to helping with migraines, apple (and other pleasing scents) can help reduce stress, reduce pain throughout the body, decrease anxiety, and even help with depression. The scent of a green apple may also be effective because of its cooling properties. It's crisp, refreshing smell is cooling (similar to mint or eucalyptus). Just as an ice pack helps reduce swelling on a sore knee, the cool scent of an apple may be reducing swelling or pressure in the brain.

If the smell of a green apple isn't particularly pleasant in your opinion, you can try other scents (like the mint or eucalyptus mentioned above) that also provide a pleasant cooling effect. If you prefer heat more than cold for pain relief, you could also try "hot" scents like cinnamon or nutmeg. If you take prescription medication to treat chronic migraines, you should definitely continue with the treatment your doctor has recommended. However, smelling an apple (or any other pleasing aroma) will not at all interfere with any prescription medication so it's perfectly safe to use as a complementary treatment.

ACTION PLAN

If your medication isn't working or you prefer to use more natural remedies, just pick up an apple and hold it to your nose. Inhale through your nose deeply and slowly. Exhale through your mouth. Repeat this, allowing the scent of the apple to fill your nose and lungs completely. You can boost the healing power of this method by slicing up some green apples and putting them in a hot bath. The heat of the water will help release the chemical compounds that produce the apple's signature scent. Green apples are used because they provide the most pungent and strong scent but if you prefer another kind of apple, you can try that one (or use a couple different varieties).

While in the bath, try using candlelight instead of the light of the bathroom. Since light can often trigger increased pain with migraines, the soft light of candles will provide a gentler glow that doesn't trigger any additional pain. The warmth of the bath itself can also help you relax and reduce pain signals in the brain. As mentioned earlier, if you don't find the scent of an apple especially pleasant, this technique may not be as effective for you. Choose another aroma that you do find pleasing. Peppermint and eucalyptus have also been shown to be highly effective in treating migraines and headaches. You can buy these scents in the form of essential oils that you just add to your bath (a few drops will do the trick) and enjoy. The important thing, no matter what scent you choose, is to focus on taking deep, slow breaths—in through your nose and out through your mouth.

In addition to just smelling the apple directly or putting it into your bath, you could also try a third method: steaming. Slice up the apples (or use essential oil) and add them to a large pot of water. Bring the water to a boil. Once boiling, pour it into another large bowl. Place your head directly over the bowl and drape a towel over your head. Again, breathe deeply and slowly through your nose and out through your mouth to inhale the scent. Do this for about 10 minutes or until the water stops producing steam. With this steaming method, you will be doubling up the pain reducing power of this treatment. Both the aroma you smell and the steam you are inhaling are working to reduce the pressure and relax you so that the pain of the migraine is alleviated.

Everyday Habit #70

Drink Chocolate Milk!

Chocolate milk is the best kind of milk but you might feel like it's a total taboo if you're trying to lose weight. However, it can actually be a great post workout boost. After an exhausting workout, your body is low on protein, carbohydrates, and key electrolytes. You need to replenish these as soon as possible in order to help your body recover and repair muscles. The electrolytes you need include calcium, potassium, and magnesium.

Milk contains a healthy dosage of all 3 of these. One cup of whole milk contains 28% of your calcium, 10% of your potassium, and 6% of your magnesium. That same cup also boasts 8 grams of protein, which is also essential after a workout. The chocolate provides a quick boost of simple carbohydrates (sugar) that will help reenergize you after the workout. It also provides additional magnesium and potassium so you're getting even more of the electrolytes your body needs. One cup of chocolate milk even provides a good portion of many essential B vitamins, which are important for your muscles and bones.

If you're still worried about the calorie count, just relax. First of all, counting calories is not the most effective way to lose weight. Making sure you get the nutrients you need and exercising regularly is the best way to burn off the extra fat. The number of calories is basically irrelevant in the end if you are focusing on eating nutritious foods. Secondly, after a workout, your metabolism is revved up and working in overdrive. It's going to burn through those calories from the milk in no time and use every last nutrient it can get from it instead of storing it as fat so you won't undo all your hard work just by indulging in a delicious, refreshing glass of chocolate milk.

ACTION PLAN

If you work out at the gym, take a bottle of chocolate milk with you. Use a well-insulated thermos to store it if there's no refrigerator available. If you work out at home, keep your fridge stocked with chocolate milk. You can also by regular whole milk and then get a chocolate mix to add to it.

In some cases, you can find chocolate mixes that are fortified with vitamins and minerals that you need. This makes it an even healthier post workout treat! Keep in mind that chocolate milk is not a substitute for water. It will help hydrate you but from all the sweating and fluid loss during that workout, you also need to drink plenty of water in addition to the milk.

The average person should be drinking at least 2 liters of water per day. If you work out, you'll need to drink more than that since you will be losing more fluid than the average person who doesn't work out. So, your post workout routine should involve a cup of chocolate milk, a tall glass of water, and maybe a banana or bowl of oatmeal. Remember, the time right after a workout is when your metabolism is at its peak so this is the best time to eat.

A good workout will also keep your metabolism elevated for a full *14 hours* after the workout so it's best to do your exercise routine first thing in the morning so you can take full advantage of this throughout the day. What better way is there to start your morning than with an invigorating workout followed by a cold glass of guilt-free chocolate milk? Well, aside from being able to sleep in, that is.

Everyday Habit #71

Something You May Not Want to Hear

So far, this book has been focusing on unique positive habits that you'll enjoy (well, with the exception of cleaning every day). This one might not sound as appealing but it's not actually as bad as it sounds so bear with me here. This habit is don't retire. Sure, you've been working hard for years and motivating yourself with the thought that eventually you'll one day retire and finally get to relax. Well, as appealing as that sounds, relaxing 24/7 is not that healthy for you. It will also get boring a lot quicker than you would imagine. Think of retirement as the opposite but equally unhealthy extreme on the other side of being in a perpetual state of high stress and anxiety.

Just as it's not healthy to *overwork* yourself, it's also not healthy to not work at all. Now, this is not to stay that you should hold down your 9 to 5 well into your golden years. You can retire from your career but do not let retirement make you inactive or sedentary. Multiple studies have shown that this kind of inactive retirement plays a huge role in senior obesity, chronic disease, and deterioration of the brain and other organs. It makes senses when you think about it. If you stop using your brain and body on a regular basis, it will fall into disuse and begin to decay—just like the old car sitting in your driveway or that abandoned building in town.

It's not flattering to think of yourself as a car or a building but if you spend your retirement sitting around "relaxing", your body and mind will start to deteriorate because they are not being used. If you stay active after retirement—getting lots of physical exercise and making sure to keep your mind engaged and working—you'll not only have a more rewarding and enjoyable retirement, you'll also have a longer retirement. Staying active will decrease your risk of obesity, dementia, Alzheimer's disease, arthritis, heart disease, stroke, diabetes, osteoporosis, and countless other diseases.

Most people mistakenly assume that these sorts of chronic illnesses are just par for the course. When you get older, things just stop working as well as they used to. While there is some truth to this, staying active (mentally and physically) can make a huge difference. It will significantly slow the process of aging and keep your body stronger and more capable of fighting off these various diseases and conditions.

ACTION PLAN

No matter what your age is now, it's never too soon (or too late) to start planning for an *active* retirement. Here are a few strategies to help you do that.

Fulfill your dreams.

You know all those plans and dreams you have but keep putting off by saying "I don't have the time"? Well, retirement is your perfect opportunity to do all of it! If you ever wanted to travel the world or learn how to swing dance, retirement is your opportunity to do it.

Help your future self out by starting a list now of all your dreams and plans that just don't seem realistic to accomplish with your current busy schedule. Call it your "Retirement To-Do List" and add to it whenever you think of something you would like to do.

Continue learning.

Staying active is just as much about keeping your mind active as it is about keeping your body active. One of the best ways to do this is to get in the habit of constantly learning new skills and gaining new knowledge.

Learn a new language. Learn how to play the guitar. Learn how to make pottery. Learn physics. There is no shortage of interesting skills and knowledge out there. Surely there is something you have always wanted to learn but never had the chance. Perhaps you always wanted to get a degree in art history or music but never could quite fit it into your schedule. Use your retirement to finally get that degree. If you've already got a degree in something else, that's even better. This time, you can focus on enjoying the courses and really absorbing the knowledge rather than stressing about grades and GPAs. If a whole degree doesn't appeal to you, you can also just sign up for interesting classes at a community college, take online courses, or just learn on your own (or with a group of friends who have similar interests).

Volunteer your time.

Volunteering is a great way to spend your retirement. Not only does it keep you active and involved in the community, it helps you to feel like you still are an important, contributing member of society (because you *are* still an important part of the community). Volunteering is also extremely rewarding. There's nothing quite like the satisfaction of knowing that *your* presence and support is improving someone's life. Find an organization or cause that you support and ask to volunteer. You could volunteer at a shelter, a school, a charity, or even a local church. There are lots of organizations out there working to make the world a better place and they depend on people like you to generously give their time to help them in that work.

Be social.

While it's not a physical illness, loneliness is an epidemic all its own among seniors. It's perfectly natural. As you get older, you start to outlive your friends and loved ones. Your children grow up and go off to start families of their own. All those familiar faces that once surrounded you slowly begin to disappear. It's easy and completely acceptable to get emotional about this. But don't let it turn you into a hermit who sits at home alone all day. Don't sulk in your misery, go out and make friends, inspire young people, and just generally stay socially active. Your life is not over once you hit your senior years. The population of seniors is growing each year, which means that you'll have plenty of people in your age group with similar experiences.

Go through the ups and downs of life as a senior together with others who are going through the exact same thing. Volunteering (which you read about above) and getting involved in sports (which you will read about next) are two great ways to be social. But you can also just go out to a bar or café. Join or start a book club or film club. Attend writing groups or workshops. Take up wine tasting and meet new people at wine tasting events. There's plenty of ways to stay social and during your retirement, you'll have plenty of time to cultivate an active and exciting social life. Who knows, it could end up being even more exciting than your social life now!

Get involved in sports.

Plan to get involved in sports and don't limit yourself to the stereotypical "old people sports" like shuffleboard or lawn bowling. Your age does not have to limit you. If you enjoy a sport and can do it without injuring yourself, go for it! You can get a head start on this one by getting involved in sports now and stick with it well into your retirement.

If you start now, you can explore different sports and see which one appeals to you most. Exercise now will also further improve your chances of avoiding the diseases and conditions of old age so that you can be sure that you will be physically capable of being just as active as you want to be in old age.

Everyday Habit #72

Surprising Benefit of Dental Hygiene

You already know that it's important to brush your teeth regularly and you probably know that you *should* be flossing regularly as well. But flossing and good dental hygiene are even more important than you could have ever imagined. A study done at New York University found that flossing daily not only reduced the risk of gum disease, it also reduced the risk of heart disease. This is likely because the bacteria in your mouth that cause gum disease also enter into your blood stream through your gums and eventually make their way into your heart, causing inflammation of the arteries and putting you at a high risk for heart disease. This study from New York University is not the only one that had such results.

Other research shows that people with a high amount of bacteria in their mouth (that is, people who don't floss or brush enough) are more likely to experience thickening of the arteries—a key sign of heart disease.

In addition to preventing heart disease, good dental hygiene can also help with the following:

- Stabilizing blood sugar levels

- Improving cognitive function (especially memory)
- Lowering the risk for infection or inflammation throughout the body
- Preventing premature birth

So, yes, your dentist is right to keep nagging you about flossing! It could do wonders for your health and wellbeing.

ACTION PLAN

It's easy to plan on flossing regularly but it's also one of those things that are hard to actually start doing. You should be flossing at least twice a day to experience the full benefits of good dental hygiene. Here are some tips to help you finally get in the habit of flossing regularly. Your dentist will be so proud!

Floss before you brush.

This is good for motivation and it also makes good sense hygienically. Brushing is (hopefully) already a habit of yours. If you brush first, there's a good chance you'll just forget to floss or lose the motivation to do it. By flossing before you brush your teeth, you can make sure that you don't forget it. Also, the act of flossing is dislodging particles and bacteria from between your teeth. But not all of it sticks to the floss. Some of it stays in your mouth. So, in order to make sure flossing is most effective, do it before you brush so that the brush can go in and sweep up the leftover particles and bacteria that didn't stick to the floss.

Set a reminder.

Since you probably brush your teeth around the same times each day, set a reminder for those times on your phone (or stick one up on your bathroom mirror if you're old fashioned) that tells you to floss. Reminders are one of the most effective ways to make sure that these important new habits don't slip your mind before they have a chance to get a foothold.

Carry floss with you.

Floss comes in small packages. It will fit easily in your purse or even in your pocket. Carry it with you so that you can floss after a meal to remove any large particles before they have a chance to spread bacteria to your teeth and gums. If you floss while you're out, try to swish some water around in your mouth afterward to clear out the loose particles and bacteria.

Everyday Habit #73

Adults Only

The last unique habit of this book might also end up being your favorite habit. This habit is to have more sex! Yes, that's right. Sex is a healthy habit—in more ways than one. So, don't let your schedule get too busy to enjoy this health-boosting activity. Sex is great for your health in so many ways. At the mental level, it is decreasing stress hormones. At the same time, it also increases dopamine and endorphins (the neurotransmitters that make you happy), which decrease depression and anxiety. In short, it's a fantastic treatment for stress, depression, anxiety and even anger issues.

At the physical level, it's providing you with a fun way to get some exercise, which burns fat, builds muscle, and strengthens your bones. Having sex at least twice a week can also boost the amount of antibodies in your immune system by 30%, which means you'll be more resilient to illness. So, if you want to avoid the cold or flu that's being passed around, jump into bed with your partner as often as you can!

It also lowers blood pressure, decreases your risk for heart attack, alleviates pain, and improves your quality of sleep. In men, it lowers the risk for prostate cancer, and in women, it improves bladder control by providing a pelvic workout that keeps your muscles down there strong.

ACTION PLAN

To enjoy the full benefits, you should be having sex at least twice a week but doing it even more often is even better! It can take away the fun if you try to strictly schedule this so avoid making it feel too much like a routine but do make a conscious effort to have sex often enough. Talk to your partner openly about sex. If you are worried that doing it too often will lead to boredom and routine, there are always ways to spice things up. Don't be afraid to try new things or explore new techniques.

Sure, they won't all be winners. Some of the new things you try will make you feel silly or start wondering why other people do it but that's no reason not to at least give it a shot. Don't be afraid to have fun and be silly in the bedroom. Sharing these kinds of experiences together will help you grow closer. They will also help both of you discover what truly excites your passion and figure out what your favorite positions and techniques are.

Even if all the new things you try don't go as planned, some of them might become your new favorites! You'll never know unless you try. Trying new things and being open with your partner will help make sure that things in the bedroom never grow stale. Your time in bed will be a guaranteed exciting time that also allows the two of you to grow closer.

If you don't have a partner at the moment or anyone that you are particularly interested in having sex with, self-stimulation will help you get some of the benefits. It won't burn as many calories or provide as dramatic of a boost to your immune system but it will still provide the mental health benefits, the lower blood pressure, the pain relief, and many of the other benefits that come with sex.

Everyday Habit #74

Weigh Yourself Regularly

Problem: I Have No Idea How to Track My Progress!

Daily, or weekly and at the same time – and record it.

It's important to weigh yourself the same time every day to make the task a routine, that way you never forget to do it. It's also important to recognize that your weight will fluctuate daily so don't get hung up on your daily weight. It can become disappointing if it appears as if the scale is never moving but just know that it takes time. You can weigh yourself weekly as long as it's always at the same time and it may give you less anxiety than watching your weight daily. Just keep at it and you will see positive results.

Don't just weight yourself!

It's easy to weigh yourself and get on with your day but the goal you should have is charting your progress. This way you can actually see the progress carry on as the weeks go by. It only takes a few seconds to do and you will wish you had after 4 weeks go by and you aren't really sure where you started and how far you have come.

One of the major key points to sticking with a goal is to be able to see results. It's easy to give up on your goal of losing weight if you can't see the progress and how far you have come.

Charting is as easy as this:

- Get a notebook and leave it on the counter or shelf by your scale
- Jump on the scale
- Record your results
- Check your goals bi-weekly or monthly to see how far you have come.

Everyday Habit #75

Plan Your Meals

Problem: I Don't Know How Many Calories I Eat in A Day!

Plan Your Meals Ahead of Time

If you are looking to lose weight planning your meals is a huge part of doing that. It may seem daunting at first to count calories but once you get the hang of things you won't even need to use the calorie counter. You need to first use a calorie counter to determine the amount of calories you need to stay at a healthy weight. If you have a particular goal in mind, for example that you want to lose one pound a week you will take your total and cut it by 500 calories.

If you want to lose weight at a slower rate than cut it by less. It can become unhealthy for you to lose more than one pound a week so it's not recommended to do so. Once you know your calorie requirements for the day you want to be able to spread those out throughout your day. For weight loss, it's best to have more small meals rather than three big meals in a day. You can break those up into 4-6 meals throughout the day. If you have a calorie requirement of 2,000 you can break them up into 4 meals of 400 calories or 6 meals of 200 calories.

Once you decide how many meals you have and how those calories can be broken up than you can decide what to eat for those 4-6 meals. It's not hard to come up with a list of meals that can be interchangeable throughout the week. A good tool to use would be the fitness app **MyFitnessPal,** which helps you to work out what foods or meals you can eat for the day. It also helps you to plan out your daily meals, which is less work for you. Your first steps should be:

- Get a calorie counter and determine your calorie requirement!
- Download MyFitnessPal to figure out meal plans
- Lose weight and be happy!

The key is to stick with your plan no matter what. You have a goal and this is part of how to reach it. Don't let yourself get off course, but if you do, get back to the plan the next day and keep going. You will get used to the plan and it will become routine, just a part of your day.

If you're enjoying this book and would love to let other potential readers know how great it is, please take a few seconds to leave a review on Amazon.com.

Everyday Habit #76

Plan & Carry Healthy Snacks

Problem: I Never Know What to Bring for Snacks!

Plan your snacks and bring them wherever you go.

A lot of people fail their diets not because of the meals but because of snack time. If you don't plan your meals ahead of time then you run the risk of grabbing a chocolate bar or a bag of chips as a midday snack. That's just going to make you fall behind on your goals. That's where planning comes in, you want to plan your snacks in the same way as you plan your meals and make sure you bring them wherever you go, whether that means to work or to the gym etc. You can continue to use MyFitnessPal to determine some great snack ideas and how to fit them into your daily plan. It's dangerous to just snack on whatever is around you because you could be eating items that are above your calorie range.

Healthy snacks are important to eat in between meals because they are going to provide you the energy you need to get through your workday. There are many great snack choices from fruits and veggies to dried fruit and nuts. The healthiest snacks you can find will contain complex carbohydrates as well as a small amount of fat and protein. So, it's important for you to really think about what you're putting into your body.

It's not just something to satisfy hunger or a craving, it's fuel for your body. Keeping to your plan is important but it's not meant to be torture either. It's okay to plan some unhealthy snacks as well as long as you don't go overboard. Depraving yourself is a great way to fail in your goals. Getting to your goal weight should be a fun adventure so try to think of it that way. Add some dark chocolate on one day and strawberries on another.

Everyday Habit #77

Find Lower Calorie Alternatives

Problem: How Can I Cut Calories Easier?

Find lower calorie alternatives

If you are looking for an easier way to cut calories you can start by looking at what you're eating. There's nothing necessarily wrong with eating a beef burger as part of your meal plan but what happens if you eat a turkey or veggie burger instead? Well your calories decrease, that's what. You can do this method with many things that you eat. It's all about taking a favorite menu item and finding out what the low-fat alternative would be. You may wonder about the taste but there's no need to worry, when it comes to burgers there are some really good ones out there that taste virtually the same if not better.

For those of you that love your french fries, why not make them fresh at home and bake them instead of frying them to avoid the fat in all that grease. You can lower calories in dairy product by buying the low-fat options instead. When getting a balanced diet, it is important to recognize that you aren't supposed to give up fat entirely, you actually need some fat in your diet to be healthy. But you should lean towards the fats that are good for you and eat them in moderation. Fat is obviously high in calories, so lowering your fat intake will help you to lose weight quickly. The more fruits and vegetables you add to your diet will also lower your calorie intake for the day. You may not know it but fruits and veggies take up a lot of room in your stomach but are low in calories. When you make a trip to the grocery store look at the other options around you. When you reach for those beef burgers look at the quality soy or turkey versions, you might surprise yourself and like them even more.

Everyday Habit #78

Eat Slowly

Problem: I've Eaten Way Too Much!

Eat your food slowly

French people are so skinny for one key reason; they really taste their food. Food to them is a delicacy in every way and when they eat, they eat slowly, savoring every bite. In doing so they also tend to not eat more than they should. The reason for this is the body needs time for the stomach to let the brain know that it's full.

If you shovel in your food and then wait to see if you are full, chances are you are overeating. We all know that sickening feeling of being too full at Thanksgiving dinner. It's all just so delicious and we fill our plates and then really enjoy ourselves. The next thing you know you're on the couch feeling like you can't move. It's because the body wasn't allowed enough time to notify the brain that all this food was coming in. Your brain did not have enough time to tell you that you were full. Eating slowly is key to watching your calorie intake for the day.

Don't scarf down your meals, instead enjoy them and then wait 20 minutes before you eat anything else. If you are still hungry at that point then it's okay to eat something else. It's not easy slowly down your eating, especially if you are hungry but it's important to not overeat.

Otherwise, you are just wasting calories that you shouldn't be eating in the first place. You will have to actually teach yourself to eat more slowly and by doing this you will find that you are full on less food!

When making a delicious dinner it can be hard not to fill your plate full with goodies. Choose instead a sensible amount of food and finish it before thinking about a second serving.

If you're still hungry you can always go back and eat more but if you fill your plate chances are you won't want to waste it and you will overeat. If you wait 20 minutes before grabbing that second plate there's a good chance you won't feel hungry.

Everyday Habit #79

Stop Drinking Calories

Problem: I Went Over My Calories!

Stop Drinking Calories

If you went over your calorie intake for the day chances are it's because you were drinking your calories. Many people when doing a plan don't incorporate drinks into their calorie intake. They then consume the same drinks throughout the day and wonder why they aren't losing weight. Your drinks have to be part of your calorie requirement so it's a good idea to drop all drinks that are high in sugar or calories. The calories that you will find in drinks such as tea, juice, booze, soda, coffee and many other drinks are huge. Especially if you are a fan of anything in a latte form at Starbucks, you might as well consider that a meal.

If you're aren't aware of how many calories are in drinks such as these than chances are you aren't realizing just how many calories you are consuming in a day on drinks alone. Many people think that juice is a healthy alternative to most other drinks but depending on the type of drink you could be consuming as many calories as a can of soda. Just because it says there is fruit in a drink doesn't make it healthy, for the most part you don't reap the benefits of the fiber of fruit and you're literally drinking in large amounts of calories.

In fact, if you just ate an orange instead of drinking orange juice you would get more nutritional value from it and you would feel fuller. The best way to get your drink on is to drink water and water alone. You can drink water all day long and not gain a pound.

If you drink it all day long you will also feel fuller and will end up eating less. Not only that but it's readily available as soon as you turn your tap on. Remove all the high calorie drinks from your fridge and start filling water pitchers. You can even infuse your water with fruit and vegetables for added flavor and more nutritional value.

Everyday Habit #80

Have Patience

Problem: I'm Not Losing Weight Fast Enough

Have some patience and think long term

Let's be honest losing weight doesn't happen overnight and it's unrealistic to think otherwise. It's just not realistic to think that you can start a diet today and lose pounds tomorrow. It takes time and that's still okay, you're still going to reach your goals. You just need a little patience. It's possible that you can lose weight quickly but that's not ideal. When you lose weight quickly you can guarantee that it's going to come back just as quickly.

The best way to lose weight is through a gradual process because then and only then will you keep it off. Losing one pound a week is realistic and healthy and that's 500 less calories a day so it's not torture on your body. If you think about losing a pound a week for 52 weeks that 52 pounds a year! How could you not be proud of that! When you focus on the goal of one pound a week it's not only achievable but it's sustainable. As you continue on with your plan there are going to be some adjustments that you have to make. You may need to add calories if you find you are eating too little or take away calories if you find that you are still consuming too many.

There will always be changes but it's important to know that you can depend on immediate results. You will just set yourself up for failure and that's the worst thing you can do when you are trying to lose weight. Just understand that it will take time and that this is a long-term goal not a short term one. Don't worry if you make a mistake and don't focus too much attention on the ups and downs, it's a process. You will see results soon enough so it's better to focus on what you look like and feel like over the next few weeks and months.

Everyday Habit #81

Aim to Exercise for Just 10 Minutes A Day

Problem: I Hate Exercising! Do I Have to Exercise?

Exercise for Just 10 Minutes.

Let me put it this way. Are you looking to lose weight for the long term? Yes? Then great, you should start considering to workout then. Especially if you are someone who wants to see results faster. A great way to get results faster is to combine exercise with nutrition. It's just science. If you work out you burn calories, it's really simple. Now, if you are someone who is very inactive or who doesn't spend a lot of time in the gym than start slow. Try just 10 minutes a day and go from there. It can be overwhelming to step into a gym and try to exercise for an hour, but 10 minutes is easy. 10 minutes can even be done at home.

Exercising is great but nutrition is where you are really going to lose the pounds. You have to change the way you eat, in order to lose weight. When it comes to exercise yes you burn calories but you can gain them back by eating unhealthy food. So, serious weight loss has to come from eating healthy meals. Having said that, you can't deny the benefits of exercising. If you combine the two you can really be unstoppable when it comes to your weight loss goals. Even if you are only burning 300 calories a day through exercise it's still 300 that you can add to the calorie count that you are burning throughout the day.

It doesn't take long to burn extra calories. If you aren't someone who wants to spend an hour in the gym than at least spend 10 minutes and see what a difference it makes. You might surprise yourself and want to stay longer. There is one thing about exercise, when you are finished you feel fantastic. Not only do you begin to feel great, you start to look great as well. You will be getting healthier and your body will begin to become toned.

Start with 10 minutes and see how it goes. You won't burn 300 calories but it's a beginning.

For the first week of your journey try 10 minutes, it doesn't matter the exercise. You can try pushups, go for a short run on the treadmill or lift some weights. Do that for a week and then increase it by 2 minutes. Continue on with that for a few months and soon enough you will be doing 30 minutes a day. That's all you will need to maintain burning 300 calories with exercise. If you choose to do more, even better!

Everyday Habit #82

Eat Real Food

Problem: I Eat Too Much Junk!

Eat real food for real results.

Have you ever heard the saying, "Abs are made in the kitchen?" It's true. You can work out as much as you want but, in the end, if you don't have a good diet you might as well forget ever having a six-pack. Whether or not that's your goal it says a lot for how important it is to eat nutritionally and avoid all that junk. The truth of the matter is people believe they get their energy from sugar and caffeine for the most part but that's only because that's all they have ever known.

If you take sugar out of your life completely and get through that dreaded sugar withdraw period you will find you have even more energy by giving your body real food. When you put real food into your body you not only look better in the long run but you begin to feel better as well. When you eat a meal, you don't get that feeling of being weighed down by your food. It can make such a huge difference in how your body feels. By eliminating processed food as well as junk food you will feel less bloated and because of that you will not only look but also feel healthier.

A good start to eating cleaner would be to begin:

- Removing junk food from your home. If you need a treat go out for ice cream instead of buying a tub of it.

- Eat more fruits and vegetables.

- Eliminate fast food and processed food.

- Limit your dairy intake.

- When it comes to grains, eat whole grain breads and rice. Limited your white starch intake.

By changing these few habits, you will make an astounding change in the way you eat. Results will come faster and you will feel better than you ever have.

Everyday Habit #83

Use Smaller Dishes

Problem: How Do I Change Eating Habits?

Use smaller dishes.

A great way to change your eating habits is by not eating as much as you used to. It will not only help to lower your calorie intake but you won't end up overeating. When you go to fill your plate, you're used to filling it up. That's what you're used to eating so you don't think anything of it. If you put less food on a big plate you notice you are eating less and it makes it that much harder to break the habit. But if you put the same smaller portion on a smaller plate you essentially trick your mind into thinking it's getting the same amount of food. This is half the battle.

Your mind isn't convinced if you put a smaller portion on the same plate you have been using for years. But change the plate and mentally it's like you are eating the same portion. Essentially when you put a smaller portion on your regular plate, your mind thinks that it's not getting enough food, even if it is. By reducing the plate size your mind thinks that everything is as it should be. You get to satisfy not only the mind but the stomach as well.

Another method you can use to minimize your portions is to eat 20% of what you would normally eat. Many people when they serve up food have the tendency to fill up bowls and set the table and allow people to feed themselves. The problem with that is when people see food in front of them they continue to eat. A good practice to keep would be to serve yourself a small portion and leave the rest at the stove.

If you are still hungry than you can get more food but chances are you will feel full with your portion and leave it at that. When you have bowls of food on the table they beckon to you to eat them and it takes a lot of self-control not to eat them. When you think about how it takes 20 minutes for your body to realize it's hungry it can be easy to get yourself into a pattern of overeating if there are bowls of food right in front of you.

Everyday Habit #84

Order Your Coffee Black

Problem: I Love Coffee! How Will I Survive?

Order your coffee black.

This may be a stretch for those that order their coffees with double or triple cream. What that means generally is that you have way too much cream and sugar in your coffee anyways. It may not be ideal for anyone to drink their coffee black but at the end of the day it's really what is best for you. When you drink your coffee black you get the caffeine benefits without the extra calories. It may surprise you to know that black coffee actually carries 0 calories. 0 calories!

That's pretty significant for a coffee drinker. So if you can manage to drink your coffee black than you are set for life. When you go to a Starbucks and grab mocha with 2% milk it has up to 260 calories which is a significant difference when you think about a black coffee having 0 calories. If you consider the possibilities of making the switch in your daily routine you are bound to lose some serious weight this year.

When you think about coffee it's clean, there's just no way around it. It's even cleaner if you can get the coffee beans and grind them yourself. Coffee isn't bad for you; the trouble comes when you start mixing cream and sugar into it. It's even worse if you add artificial sweeteners into the mix. You are adding unnecessary sugar into your diet when you mix things with your coffee and tea; sugar you don't need in your diet. The problem with sweeteners is that, not only are you adding sugar that isn't needed but you are also adding dangerous chemicals ingredients that should never be in your body to begin with.

May lattes are loaded with sugar, which makes any of those types of drinks extremely unhealthy for you to drink. Your best bet is to drink black coffee or unsweetened tea. If you are dead set against drinking your coffee black then there are things that you can try. You have the option of making your own almond milk coffee creamer. It takes some time but if you are open to it than it may be a better alternative to black coffee.

Everyday Habit #85

Make Walking After Dinner A Habit

Problem: It's Hard to Be Motivated After a Meal!

Make walking after dinner a habit!

What do you usually do after dinner? Go sit in front of the TV and vegetate for the rest of the evening? What usually happens after that is you hit the hay. You're exhausted after all from a long day and that's all you want to do. That's not usually the best idea even if all you want to do is relax. But what you need to do is think about what is really going on in your body. After you eat, food is being digested. Your blood sugar levels are going up...after that fat levels are rising in your blood vessels.

The best thing that you can do for yourself at this point is to think about your health, and really all that does is take 15 minutes. Instead of heading for the TV what you need to do is head for your front door. Studies have shown that when you walk after meals especially a heavy dinner it can help you to lower your blood sugar as well as your triglyceride levels. If that isn't reason enough to go for a walk then you have to consider the facts that it improves your digestion, burns calories and overall helps you lose weight.

There are many benefits to walking after a meal:

- **Lowers triglycerides** - triglycerides affect your cardiovascular health, and promote heart attacks. Studies show that exercise suppresses triglycerides. But this doesn't give you the right to gorge on a heavy meal and then go for a walk; it just doesn't work that way.

- **Lower Blood Sugar** - Your weight and diet have a huge role in how much weight you gain, not only that but you could be at risk for diabetes. Studies have shown that overweight people who walk for 15 minutes after a meal showed an improved daily blood sugar level. That blood sugar level improved the more the person walked.

- **Faster Digestion** - Everyone feels full after a meal. The great thing about walking after a meal is that you digest your food faster.

- **You burn calories** - If you walk at a decent pace for 15 minutes after a meal you are likely to burn about 60 calories which is nothing to sneeze at.

Below are some tips to motivating yourself to walking after dinner:

1. **Walk with a partner**

Make a pact with your spouse or even a friend to walk after dinner. There is accountability there if one of you tries to drop out.

2. **Take your Dog**

Make it a habit of taking your dog for a walk after dinner. This way you kill two birds with one stone.

3. **Associate Walking with Sleep**

If you take a walk after dinner chances are that you will sleep a lot better that night. So if you are looking for a good night's rest than consider the benefits of walking after dinner.

Everyday Habit #86

Eat Salad Dressing On The Side

Problem: I love Salad Dressing!

Eat salad dressing on the side.

It's not hard to see why you should order salad dressing on the side. Typically, when you are at a restaurant and you order salad you get salad soaked with dressing, more than you even need. The problem with that is you are eating calories that are totally unnecessary. You can enjoy a salad with dressing without going overboard.

Whether you know it or not dressing is high in calories. The only way to control those calories is by ordering it on the side and adding just what you need. You have a few choices, you can either dip your fork into the salad dressing or proceed in that manner or you can add a tablespoon to your salad and eat it like that.

If you need to add more you can, but you have complete control over how much salad dressing you consume. Be smart about eating especially when you are at a restaurant. They don't think about serving people who are on a diet. They serve a lot of food for the most part to keep customers happy.

If you are on a diet a restaurant is typically a bad place to be in. It doesn't mean that you can't eat out ever but help yourself as much as possible when you are out. If you are at home there are many salad dressings you can make at home that don't have the added preservatives and sugar that the store made ones do. This will also help to eliminate extra calorie intake.

Everyday Habit #87

Stop Ordering Appetizers & Desserts

Problem: I Love Ordering Desserts After Dinner!

Stop ordering appetizers and desserts!

Appetizers can be tantalizing and delicious when you are looking over them on a menu. And they are! But more often than not you don't need them and they only lead to overeating. The problem with appetizers is that they are only on the menu to satisfy restaurant owners. They are added to the menu to bring in extra profit and they do. But for the customer all they bring in is extra calories. Appetizers are literally the worst things to order from a restaurant menu and the only thing worse than an appetizer is a dessert. No one goes to a restaurant to be hungry after a meal so chances are you are already full after your meal or well on the way.

When you order a dessert, you are just adding on extra calories that you don't even need. You are already full and yet you are willing to add those extra calories just for the sake of ordering a dessert to fill a craving. When it comes to deciding what to eat avoid the appetizer. Don't order them at all, just don't do it. They are just the worst things to order. They become even worse if you order them without any intention of sharing them with anyone.

If you can't help yourself and you just need to order something sweet after your meal there are ways around it without compromising your diet completely. Order a dessert and only take 3 bites. It may sound silly but all you need is a few bites to curb a craving, you don't have to eat an entire piece of cake. If you feel you might be caving in this is your best bet, enjoy three bites guilt-free and then move the plate to the other side of the table and stay focused on your diet.

Everyday Habit #88

Eat Before You Get Really Hungry

Problem: Sometimes I'm Starving Before I Ever Begin Eating!

Eat before you get really hungry!

The worst thing you can do is wait to eat until you are very hungry. We all do it, whether it is a long day at work or we get caught up doing too many tasks, there are times that we don't eat when we should. If we wait too long we get desperately hungry and then at that point we will eat just about anything. If we get too hungry we have the habit of eating really terrible choices just because it's convenient for us.

Not only that but we also tend to eat too fast and we end up eating too much. We are so hungry that we are trying to rid ourselves of that feeling as quickly as possible so we eat a lot of food in a short period of time. The next thing we know we are overeating and that's the worst thing you could do if you're trying to lose weight. It's best to not put off eating until you get to the point where you are starving.

Here are a few quick tips to help you to eat less and spot hunger before it gets to the starving stage. Not only will you be able to control your calorie intake but you will also be able to shed pounds. There is a hunger scale that can help you recognize what hunger really feels like. Learn to recognize your physical cues so you know when you actually need nourishment and when you are just having a craving.

Before you eat, use the hunger scale below to determine what you really need:

1. **Starving:** It's that very uncomfortable empty feeling you get that is often accompanied by a light-headed feeling. You may also experience the jitters, they are caused by a low blood sugar level due to lack of food. If you are this hungry the chances of you binging are very high.

2. **Hungry:** You are thinking about your next meal. You have about an hour before you enter the starving category if you do not eat something.

3. **Moderately Hungry:** At this point you may be experiencing growling in your stomach. You may be thinking of putting an end to your hunger. This would be the perfect time to sit down and eat your meal.

4. **Satisfied:** You're not full but you aren't hungry either. You feel comfortable and relaxed, you aren't necessarily thinking about eating.

5. **Full:** At this point if you are still eating, it's due to momentum and nothing else. You are no longer hungry you

just like the taste of the food. You may start to feel slightly bloated but the food begins to not taste as good as it did when you were hungry.

6. **Stuffed:** This is the point when your body feels uncomfortable. You may even experience some mild heartburn from your stomach acids creeping back to your esophagus.

Everyday Habit #89

Always Pack Your Lunch

Problem: Brown Bag Lunches Are Boring!

Always pack your lunch when trying to lose weight!

We're not talking about peanut butter and jam sandwiches here; you can have great lunches prepared at home for a fraction of the cost for eating out at lunch. Not only that but you can control the calories you intake. When you make a lunch at home you know what's going into your body. If you grab a lunch on the go chances are you are going to end up with an unhealthy alternative and it will most likely be high in calories. You will be eating better food when you pack a lunch from home but not only that you are also guaranteeing that you don't miss or skip your lunch if you get too busy during the day.

Your lunch will already be there for you to nibble on while you work instead of worrying about having to leave the office to go and grab something. It's so much easier to find lunch from your own fridge than it is to go out and try to decide what to have for lunch. If you know you are going to be away from home for lunch than save yourself some time and money by packing a lunch from home.

Many foods can be taken for lunch that doesn't need to be refrigerated such as cooked legumes, fruits and veggies, as well as certain grains. If you want to take meat, dairy or eggs it's pretty easy to pick up an insulated container to bring your lunch in.

There are many different options for you to take healthy lunches to work; here are just a few ideas:

- Soup with vegetables and legumes, such as black beans, lentils or chickpeas. Pair that with a green salad and some light dressing.

- Leftovers are great for lunches. A leftover stir-fry with vegetables, brown rice and tofu is just the kind of healthy lunch you need.

- Sandwiches are always a common choice. Make sure you add some veggies and pair it with an orange and some baked black bean tortilla chips.

- Pita bread with lean turkey, sprouts, and cranberry sauce. Bring low-fat yogurt or Greek yogurt as a sweet treat.

- Pair oat bran bread with turkey breast, green pepper rings and tomato slices for a delicious sandwich. Add a piece of fruit and some yogurt and you're set.

- Vegetarian chili, wheat crackers, carrots and an apple.

- Cheese and apple slices on a pita. Bring more fruit and a yogurt.

Everyday Habit #90

Deal with Stress

Problem: Is Stress Affecting How I Lose Weight?

You need to deal with your stress if you hope to lose weight.

Life can be stressful and oftentimes hard to avoid. But the level of stress you are experiencing can actually affect whether or not you can lose weight. If you have a stressful career or happen to be in a relationship that has more downs than ups stress can affect your body in ways you never knew. Some people deal with stress by overeating, which could be detrimental to your health as well as make it hard to be on any type of diet. If you have stressful things going on in your life you need to either deal with the stress or change the situation so that you no longer have that stress in your life. Not only is stress bad for your health it's bad for your life in general.

Unfortunately for most of us stress is just a way of life. The downside to that is that stress is also what can make you fat. Even if you eat well and exercise, stress can make it hard for you to lose weight. It doesn't just make it hard to lose weight it can actually add more pounds to you. When you are stressed out your brain tells your cells to release potent hormones. When this happens, you get an adrenaline rush that taps into your stored energy. At the same time that this happens you get a surge of cortisol that tells your body you need to replenish energy even if you haven't used up your stored fat. If this happens you feel hungry, very hungry even if you have recently eaten something. Your body will continue producing the cortisol that makes you feel hungry as long as you are stressed out. What makes it worse is that when this happens, we rarely grab veggies, instead we go for the salty snacks or the sweets. We seek these things out because they make us feel better when we are stressed. Every time you feel stressed you seek out these comfort foods and then it becomes one big viscous cycle.

When your body is producing cortisol, it stops producing testosterone, which helps you build muscle. So not only are you putting on pounds but they are also not being turned into muscle. When there is a drop-in muscle building than you burn fewer calories. It's important to reflect on what is making you stressed and eliminate it or lessen the stress from your life. It's the best thing for you. Meditation or Yoga are both great ways of relieving stress and thinking positively.

Everyday Habit #91

Sit Down to Eat

Problem: Sometimes I Have to Eat On The Go!

It's important to sit down and eat rather than eating and running.

When we are running out the door with food in our hands we aren't really focusing on the task of eating. We are focusing on getting to work or running an errand. By not focusing on eating we can end up overeating or grabbing something unhealthy as we head out the door. What you want to do is actually sit down and eat. Take your time and really focus on what you are eating. This is going to allow you to have a healthy meal and it may even help you to decrease your stress level.

That's the rule: Sit down and eat. An exception to this rule could be snacking but even them you should sit down and focus on what you are eating as much as possible.

Everyday Habit #92

Cut Down Your TV Time

Problem: I Love Watching TV While I Eat!

Cutting down your TV time is very important.

You're not alone, everyone likes to sit in front of the TV and relax while eating. It's a common practice especially after a long day at work, sometimes you just want to zone out for a while. Everybody loves a good dose of TV to get the relaxing started. TV to an extent though has a lot of control over our lives. We can easily let life pass us by if we spend all our time glued to a couch watching TV. We indulge in meaningless programs and watch food commercials, which, by the way, make us want to eat. The problem with that is we are so focused on the TV that we aren't focused on how much we eat and that's where overeating can come in. Turn off the TV, finish your meal and get outside!

Everyday Habit #93

Eat on A Schedule

Problem: Does It Matter When I Eat?

Eating on a schedule is key to losing weight.

The best thing about having a routine is that it forces you not to stray in areas that are going to get you off your goals. It's no different when you set up an eating schedule. When you have an eating schedule ready to go it forces you to be more conscious of planning your meals ahead of time. That way you are never rushed and making bad food choices. If everything is planned out then it's easier to keep that metabolic rate in check and you won't have to worry about getting hungry and having your blood sugar spike. A good plan should be to eat every three hours during the day. You may not like being on a schedule especially if you are used to flexibility but stick with it. Being structured in this area will keep you from making bad food choices when you're hungry.

Everyday Habit #94

Keep A Food Diary

Problem: I Keep Forgetting to Write My Food Down!

Keep a food diary helps you make proper food choices.

The first time a trainer told me to keep a food diary I thought to myself, what is the point? How is this going to help me lose weight? But it will and it's a great tool to use to determine how much food you actually consume in a day. Most people have no idea how much food they eat in a day. That can be a dangerous game to play because you may be downing more calories than you need.

Another option you may find is that you aren't eating enough calories. It can work both ways but if you keep a food diary you will know how many calories you are eating and can adjust as you go along. By tracking the food you eat you can also make better eating choices. You may realize that you aren't making the best choices and can change your eating habits. It also holds you accountable to what you are putting into your body.

Keep a record of what you eat for breakfast, lunch and dinner as well as the snacks and drinks you consume throughout the day. You may be surprised what you find out while keeping the diary.

Everyday Habit #95

Opt for The Stairs

Problem: Any Suggestions for Losing Extra Calories?

Try taking the stairs!

Sounds too easy, right? But you would be surprised how many people avoid taking the stairs at work at all cost. It's just so much easier to jump on the escalator or get in the elevator but you can make a huge difference in your weight loss by taking the stairs every single day. It may be hard to do at first but after a while it's not going to feel hard at all and you will be burning extra calories in a very easy way.

Everyday Habit #96

Park Further from The Door

Problem: I Like to Park as Close as I Can So I Can Get into Work on Time!

Leave a little earlier in the morning and park further from the door.

Everyone is usually in a hurry in the morning to get to work and we can even be sluggish in doing so. So, set your alarm for ten minutes earlier and park further from the door. Walking will not only help you burn off calories but it will wake you up a bit and give you some more energy for your day. It's a quick and easy way to incorporate a little bit of exercise in your day especially if you aren't going to the gym. A little each day will make a difference.

Everyday Habit #97

Never Skip Meals

Problem: Sometimes I Avoid Eating Breakfast!

It's important to never skip any meals.

This is an important note to be making; you absolutely must never skip meals even if you are really busy. It can be really easy to walk out the door in the morning without breakfast because you slept in or skip lunch if you are busy at the office but it's really the worst thing you could do. If you starve your body of food it will actually signal a starvation mode in your brain that tells your body that you are starving and to start storing fat. Believe me, that's the last thing you want to happen when you are trying to lose weight. It's important to make time for your meals to keep yourself healthy and to stay on track to losing weight.

Everyday Habit #98

Slow Down with The Carbs

Problem: I Love Carbs!

When thinking of weight loss, it's important to cut out a lot of carbs.

When you want to lose weight a low carb diet is the best way to do that. You need real food that is unprocessed with low carbs. Not only will you lose weight on a low carb diet but you will also become healthier and prevent the risk of developing certain disease.

The kind of foods you eat depends on how much weight you want to lose. Here is a general guideline of what you can eat:

Things to Eat

- Vegetables
- Fruit
- Meat
- Eggs
- Seeds
- Fats
- Healthy oils
- Nuts
- Non-gluten grains

Things You Don't Eat

- Sugar
- Artificial sweeteners
- Diet or low-fat products
- Trans fats
- Wheat
- Seed oils
- Processed foods

Everyday Habit #99

Less Meat, More Grains & Vegetables

Problem: How Do I Give Up Meat?

You don't need to give it up, just eat less meat.

This can be something hard to do if you're a heavy meat-eater. It can also be a task if you are used to meals that are high in meat and potatoes but it can be done. You don't have to cut it out entirely but don't eat it in excess either. You don't need to eat 8 ounces of meat at every meal; your body doesn't need it. A serving of 2-4 ounces is plenty of meat and if you combine it with some grains and vegetables you will be more than full.

Everyday Habit #100

Start Eating Soup Regularly

Problem: What's Great for Lunch?

Soup is a meal that you should have regularly.

I'm not talking about buying canned soup from a store; those cans have way too much sodium and very little flavor to them. I'm talking about making your own delicious and flavorful soup. It's perfect because you can make a large batch and freeze it for later. You will always have food on hand.

It's not usually any more than 30 minutes of prep work before your soup begins to cook. You let the soup simmer for a few hours and have a delicious meal. If you load the soup up with plenty of vegetables you will be more than full.

Others who are considering purchasing this book would love to know what you think. If you could spare a few seconds, they would greatly appreciate reading an honest review from you. Simply visit the page on Amazon.com.

Everyday Habit #101

Don't Bring Junk Food Home

Problem: How Do I Avoid Junk Food?

A good way to avoid it is to not bring it home.

Most people have bags of chips or cookies in their cupboard; you're certainly not the only one. There's ice cream in the freezer and dips in the fridge and it can be hard to avoid the temptation of those things. It's best to clear out all the junk and avoid bringing it home at all. You are bound to cheat if it's sitting there and you find yourself hungry and looking for a snack.

So, take an hour and go through your cupboards and throw away anything that's going to tempt you. You can't eat it if it isn't around and if you ever need to treat yourself you can go out for a treat. That way it's just a onetime thing instead of having a huge tub of ice cream just waiting for you.

Everyday Habit #102

Always Shop with A Full Belly

Problem: Sometimes I Shop When I'm Hungry!

Make sure you are full when you make a trip to the grocery store.

The worst thing you can do is go shopping while hungry, you will end up making some really bad food choices. Not only that but you tend to snack on unhealthy food while you shop.

Don't go in a grocery store without a plan. Make a list before you head out so that you know exactly what you are looking for. Without a list, you will start wandering the aisles and end up purchasing more than you needed to. Those extra purchases always tend to be junk food.

By having a list your impulse shopping is put to a minimum. You want to stock only healthy food in your cupboards and fridge.

More Bonus Tips!

Do you want to get the best out of life – starting today?

These are some extra awesome tips, some are similar to previous ones (just to emphasize how important I believe they are).

Living your best possible life means adopting healthier habits so that your body is in the best shape possible to handle what life throws at you. This chapter is going to teach you what you need to do in order to get on the path to wellbeing. Each part will teach you about a different habit to adopt and tell you why you should adopt that habit. There are 24 habits in total (including the bonus ones!).

I realize that 24 sounds like a lot but the trick to getting through all of them is to adopt only 1 at a time. When you have that 1 habit in the bag, then you can move on to the next one.

I suggest that you start off either by reading the whole book or, at least, scanning the various chapters. Because each of us is different, we all have different priorities. The beauty of this book is that you can basically pick and choose the order in which you will adopt the habits. You may find that some of the habits are easier to adopt than others – you can start with those if you want to. As you progress, you will feel healthier and more easily able to cope with the habits that you find harder to adopt. Just make sure that you take it nice and slowly – it may be tempting to try and take on everything at once but that is not likely to be sustainable. Rome wasn't built in a day – reversing a lifetime of bad habits is a lot easier if you take one small step at a time.

Everyday Habit #103

Don't Retire

"Evidence shows that in societies where people stop working abruptly, the incidence of obesity and chronic disease skyrockets after retirement," says Luigi Ferrucci, director of the Baltimore Longitudinal Study of Aging. He goes on to cite research done in Italy's Chianti region, where there are a large proportion of centenarians.

Pensioners there never really stop working – after retirement, they concentrate on farming vegetables or grapes. The key is that they get out and about every day and are physically active. According to a study conducted by Josef Zweimuller of the University of Zurich, early retirement can shorten your lifespan by as much as two months for every year that you retire early. Researchers put that down to a more sedentary lifestyle after retirement.

Retirement can be a big adjustment to make – after working for somewhere close to 40 years, you cannot just abruptly stop and do nothing. This sets you up to develop depression. It may not feel like it but work is a very social activity and that is another reason why you should find something else to do after retirement – something that allows you to socialize as well. If gardening is not something that appeals to you, you can always look for something else – even if that means volunteering.

Get Out and About

Many charitable organizations welcome volunteers. Alternatively, see if you can help out at your local library or museum. If you want a chance to shape young minds, the **Experience Corps** is an interesting program that allows volunteers to help out at public schools for a few hours a week, allowing them to pass on the wealth of experience they have garnered over time to the youth.

ACTION PLAN

- Think about activities that you enjoy and that you would be able to incorporate into your day after retirement.

- List your skills and experience.

- Find opportunities that allow you to bring your experience to bear and that allow you to socialize and be active.

- Remember that you are only as old as you feel – stop acting your age. Act like a kid again if it makes you feel younger and more vibrant.

Everyday Habit #104

Get At Least 6 Hours of Sleep

Ferrucci has also found that sleep is essential when it comes to the regulation and healing of cells. Getting enough sleep is vital to well-being; it's as important as diet and exercise. The optimal minimum amount of sleep is six hours for adults. Getting less than this means that you are probably short-circuiting the healing REM phases of sleep.

It is in REM phase where the body repairs itself – getting too little REM sleep means that your body is less able to repair itself and more likely to show signs of aging and disease. Getting enough sleep is actually fairly easy. It is just a matter of listening to your body's own natural rhythm.

Good Sleep Habits

Sleeping can become a habit – you can train your body when to sleep and when to wake. What you need to do is to get into a routine. To start off with, you need to get up at the same time every morning. Ideally you should be able to wake up without having to rely on your alarm clock.

If you are getting enough sleep, your body will automatically wake at around about the same time every day. If you need to rely on an alarm clock for the moment, that is fine. You just need to remember the cardinal rule – set it for the same time every day, no matter what time you went to bed the night before. You also need to learn to ignore the snooze button.

By sleeping late some days, you are disturbing the body's own sleep/wake cycle making it more likely that you will have problems getting a good night's rest throughout the week. By the same token, you should aim to go to sleep at around about the same time every night. After a few weeks, your body will learn this new rhythm and it will become automatic.

Good Sleep Hygiene

Good sleep hygiene will make it easier to fall asleep and to stay asleep. You should switch off all electronic devices such as your TV, computer, etc. at least an hour before bedtime. If possible, dim the lights around about this time as well.

The artificial lights can interfere with melatonin production. Melatonin is a hormone that makes you sleepy and is produced naturally by the body.

Working on your computer or watching TV can be very stimulating and can leave your mind racing making sleep next to impossible. By switching off these items an hour before bedtime, you are signaling your body that it is time to start winding down for the night. Use the time to relax – read for a bit or take a warm bath. This allows your body and mind a chance to relax.

A quick cheat is to wear sunglasses in the evening to help reduce the amount of light that you see and to help trick your body into producing melatonin. Another tip is to steer clear of all stimulants after 2pm. Tea, coffee, sodas, etc. generally contain caffeine and sugar and the effects of these stimulants can be felt for hours after you have consumed them.

Getting enough exercise will help you to sleep better at night, as long as you do not exercise within 4-6 hours of bedtime. Exercising in the evening can rev up your metabolism and make it more difficult to fall asleep. You also need to make sure that your bedroom is primed as a haven for sleeping in. Banish the TV and make sure that you never take work to bed with you. Your mind should associate your bed primarily with sleep – that way the very act of climbing into bed will help you to feel sleepy.

Your bedroom should be as uncluttered and orderly as possible. It should be soothing rather than bright. You need to make sure that it is as dark as possible at night – using thick curtains or blackout blinds can go a long way to this end. LED displays are a bad idea – they give off a lot of light and this can interfere with sleep. Clock radios are amongst the worst culprits but any LED light, even a small stand-by light can make a difference.

The room should be well-ventilated and comfortably cool in order for you to sleep well. Your bed should be comfortable and firm enough to support you. Buy the best quality bed linen that you can afford – of all-natural materials if possible. Natural materials allow skin to breathe making it easier for your body to regulate its own temperature. Your core body temperature drops when sleeping so you should ensure that you have enough warm blankets where applicable. It is especially important to make sure that your feet are warm enough as cold feet can cause sleep disturbances.

Hello Darkness My Old Friend

Too much external light can keep you awake at night. Make sure that your curtains cut out as much light as possible. Angling your bed away from the windows so that the light is not shining directly on your face can also help. In need, wear a sleeping mask. If you live in a warmer area, look for one made out of toweling or natural fabrics – synthetic ones will not allow the skin to breathe and can make you feel hot, sweaty and uncomfortable.

Controlling the Noise

Something as simple as crickets chirping could drive you nuts if you are battling to sleep. Traffic noises or dogs barking could also interfere with sound sleep. If you live in a noisy area, consider wearing earplugs. Get the more comfortable soft silicone types that fit into your ear snugly to cut out most noises.

Skip the Sleeping Pills

Sleeping pills can be used as a short-term measure but care must be taken, as they are highly addictive. Use them only as a last resort and never for longer than a week at a time. While they will help you to fall asleep earlier, the sleep will be lighter and less refreshing.

Natural herbal supplements such as Valerian and Passion Flower can be a valuable aid if you are having trouble sleeping but, again, you should not use them over long periods. A cup of warm chamomile tea can help you to relax and feel sleepy. A glass of warm milk can help in a similar way.

Don't Make Mountains Out of Molehills

The very worst thing that you can do is to toss and turn in bed worrying about how little sleep you are getting. If you do not fall asleep within 20 minutes, you have two choices:

- Get up out of bed and do something else. Preferably something that won't stimulate your mind too much. Sit and read until you start to feel drowsy, for example. Do not switch the TV or computer on and stop watching the clock.

- Stay in bed and relax. The very act of lying still in your bed will do your body some good so there is no need to be concerned about sleep as well.

  You need to be able to let worrying about sleep go – if you fall asleep, great, if not, it is not the end of the world.

When you are battling to fall asleep, it may feel like the most desperate situation in the world. Studies have shown though that we sleep more than we realize – you may even nod off now and then and not realize that you have slept at all. Your body should eventually right itself – you may have a couple of sleepless nights and then find yourself crashing the third night.

Get to the Root of the Problem

If you find that you have chronic insomnia that goes on for longer than a week, you should go and see your doctor to rule out physical causes. Unbalanced blood sugar and diabetes can cause sleep issues so it is important to rule these out. Depression and anxiety may also cause sleep disturbances so get yourself checked out for these as well.

Live a Healthier Lifestyle

Unfortunately, you mother was right here – eating all your veggies and getting enough exercise and fresh air is important for your health and sleep. You need to find ways to actively manage your stress levels and to live a healthier lifestyle if you are dealing with chronic insomnia.

ACTION PLAN

- Go to your bedroom and clear out any unnecessary clutter. Make your bedroom a calm sanctuary.

- Get rid of the TV in the bedroom, if applicable. Keep your laptop out of it as well. Make sure that your phone is on bedside mode, if it has one and avoid charging the phone when you are sleeping. (Some phones light up when charging and this could interfere with sleep).

- After lights out tonight, check for appliances that give off light or make a noise and check whether or not your curtains let in a lot of light.

- If necessary, measure your windows and get blackout blinds.

- Look for music that soothes and relaxes you. Music can be great at distracting the mind from the fact that you are unable to sleep and can put you in a more relaxed frame of mind.

- Practice visualization techniques to clear your mind – imagine a huge blackboard and then watch as a white dot appears. Imaging the dot expanding until the whole board is white. Then imagine a black dot on the white board and repeat the visualization until you fall asleep.

- Deep breathing can help you to relax and fall asleep. Concentrate on your breathing and inhale deeply to a count of four, all that matters is the counting, nothing else. Hold your breath for a count of four, again concentrating on the counting before exhaling to the count of four. Repeat until you feel sleepy.

Everyday Habit #105

MOVE!

"Exercise is the only real fountain of youth that exists," says Jay Olshansky, a professor of medicine and aging researcher at the **University of Illinois at Chicago**.

"It's like the oil and lube job for your car. You don't have to do it, but your car will definitely run better." Countless studies have proven that exercise benefits mood, balance, mental fitness, bone density and muscle mass.

"And the benefits kick in immediately after your first workout," Olshansky adds.

And you don't need to be a gym addict to see benefits – in fact, those who get the most benefit are those people who give up the sedentary lifestyle and just walk around the block or the nearest shopping mall. 30 minutes a day is all that you need to improve your health.

Building muscle with resistance training or yoga will enable you to build muscles that are leaner and more toned and help to convert flab to muscle. This, in turn, will help you to fight the effects of middle age spread – as we age, our metabolism slows down. From middle age onwards, if not counteracted, this can mean an increase in weight of a couple of pounds a year. Our bodies were not designed to live a sedentary life – if you want to be in the best health possible, you should be getting at least half an hour of cardiovascular exercise daily.

Worried that you don't have the time? Fortunately, the most up to date research shows that the effect of exercise is cumulative so you do not have to do 30 minutes in a row. You can, if it is easier to do so, break this up into 3 x 10-minute sessions. You will achieve the same benefit and it will be a lot easier to fit in the sessions.

What could be easier? A quick 10-minute walk before breakfast, a 10-minute walk during your lunch break and a quick walk when you get home in the evening and your exercise for the day is done. Exercise can be a cheap and easy way for you to maximize your weight loss efforts. You just need to kick up your feet and stop making excuses – get moving now.

Exercise in the Morning

To really amp up the benefits, you should schedule an exercise session first thing in the morning, before eating breakfast, as soon as possible after getting out of bed.

If possible, exercise in full sunlight so that your body wakes up completely. Exercise revs up your metabolism for 4-6 hours after you have finished. Boosting your metabolism as early as possible in the morning means that you are able to get the full advantage of the boost. By exercising before breakfast, you are forcing your body to rely on its own internal energy stores, thereby revving up fat burning. Your body has no food that it can draw on for energy so it needs to access the fat.

If you are aiming to lose weight, exercising before breakfast is one of the legitimate shortcuts that you can take to maximize your fat-burning efforts. Scheduling your exercise for earlier in the day also increases the likelihood that you will get the exercise done. If it is over and done with first thing in the morning then there are no quick "emergencies" that can crop up later in the day.

We've all been there – we get out of bed and the day looks brighter; we eat a wonderful, healthy breakfast and are sure that we are going to have a healthy day. Then disaster strikes at work – you need to fix a big mistake, your own, or someone else's and suddenly the world doesn't look as great anymore.

You leave work late and are fed up by the time you get home. You decide to can the exercise and dig into the ice cream instead. We have all been there. Your motivation to exercise is likely to be at its highest point in the morning before the stresses of the day take their toll – start your day with exercise and you reduce the amount of excuses that you can make.

What Exercise?

Anything that gets your heart rate up is going to do you some good. There is no need to half-kill yourself while exercising either. Rather start off at a slower pace that you can manage and work your way up from there. That way, you will be less likely to injure yourself and will be more likely to make exercise a habit going forward. Once it is a habit, you will start to look forward to your daily sessions.

If you are pretty unfit, you need to consider a low impact exercise that is easy to incorporate into your daily schedule. Both walking and swimming provide an easy way to get your heart rate up without putting too much stress on your body. At the end of the day though, anything that gets your body moving will help – if you find something that you enjoy doing, it is even better. The more you enjoy exercising, the less it will feel like a chore and the more likely you will be to continue with it.

Exercise can take many forms – formal exercise such as aerobics; dancing; washing the car; etc. Anything that gets your heart rate up will do. You can use the exercise time to play with your kids – have you ever tried keeping up with a toddler or small kiddy? They are bundles of energy. Alternatively, you can start walking the dog. This is great exercise for both of you and also a great way to bond with your dog. Walking them can help to relieve boredom for them as well.

Your Heart Rate and You

Monitor your heart rate to ensure that you keep in the fat-burning zone. If you do not have a heart monitor, all you need to do is to measure your pulse for 10 seconds. Multiply that total by 6 and you will know what your heart rate is. You want to keep at an activity level that gets you to about 80% of your maximum heart rate. This is the optimal rate for fat burning.

Your maximum heart rate is easy to work out. All you need to do is to subtract your age from 220. Work out what 80% of that figure is and you have your target rate to work on. It can also be helpful to take your resting pulse rate every morning to see how you are progressing in terms of fitness. The fitter you are, the slower your pulse. A slower pulse rate is worth aiming for – it means that your heart is not having to work as hard and is more efficient at circulating your blood. A person in reasonably good shape will have a resting heart rate in the 60's.

Now Stretch!

Add in a five-minute stretch routine before each session so that your muscles are properly warmed up and follow the same routine after exercising to ensure that the muscles are cooled down. Stretching has benefits of its own. It helps to prepare the muscles for a workout in a gentle way and so help to prevent injury.

It can help to make the muscles look longer and leaner and will help the body to remove lactic acid from the muscles. The muscles produce lactic acid when they are doing work that they are not accustomed to and it is the lactic acid that makes you feel stiff and sore in the days after you exercise. As you get more used to exercising, this soreness will pass. A few years ago it was very popular to do the bouncing stretch. This has since been proven to be counter-productive. Rather concentrate on getting a good solid stretch in and maintaining the right form.

Strengthen your Body

At some point you will also need to look at some form of strength training in order to reshape your body. For the ladies worried that this is going to make them look like Mr. Universe, out those fears aside – women are not naturally able to look that ripped, it takes a lot of work and careful dieting to look like that. If you are following a normal strength-training program, you can expect to look leaner and feel stronger, nothing more than that.

Strength training sessions are best broken up into upper body sessions and lower body sessions. Never work the same parts of the body two days in a row – your muscles need time to rest and repair in between. You could do lower body exercises on Monday, Wednesday and Friday and upper body exercises on Tuesday, Thursday and Saturday, for example.

There is no need to invest in tons of specialized equipment either – start by trying out different forms of exercise until you settle on one or two that you enjoy – then you can buy the equipment.

Find a Partner in Crime

Having an exercise buddy can be a great way to motivate you to exercise. Choose someone who is around about the same fitness level as you. There are two advantages here – when doing aerobic exercise, you should aim for a level that raises the heart rate but that still allows you to carry a conversation. You and you buddy can thus chat while going for a walk – it will make the time seem to go faster.

In addition, being held accountable by someone else for exercising can be truly motivating. Often when we are on our own it is a lot easier to blow off exercise and do something else. If you know that your buddy is relying on you to see it through, you are less likely to come up with an excuse to skip on the exercise.

ACTION PLAN

- List the sports/ games activities that you used to enjoy as a kid – is there a form of exercise out there that can match? Look for something that is fun.

- List three ideal time zones that you can set aside for exercise starting tomorrow – this might mean getting out of bed 15 minutes earlier or taking a pair of sneakers to work – look for ways that you can incorporate more exercise instead of excuses as to why you cannot.

- Go to your local library and see what exercise DVD's they have or are able to order for you. Alternatively, go to your local fitness store and see if any there appeal to you.

- Check out your local gym and see whether or not there are trial memberships on offer – do not get pressured into signing a contract, try it out before you commit.

- Get more exercise today by making smarter decisions – park your car further away from the door at the mall or from your office and walk the rest of the way. Is it feasible for you to walk or cycle to the shops or work?

Everyday Habit #106

Start Jogging

The great thing about jogging is that you can do it anywhere – all you need is a decent pair of shoes. Danish researchers have actually found that jogging is the best exercise when it comes to extending your life.

"We can say with certainty that regular jogging increases longevity," researcher Peter Schnohr said in a release. "The good news is that you don't actually need to do that much to reap the benefits." Schnohr found that jogging between 1 and 2 ½ hours a week could add another 6 years to our life expectancy. That is less than the ½ an hour a day recommended for cardiovascular health!

We know about the **immediate benefits of exercise** like the so-called runner's high – where the body releases endorphins in response to exercise – but there are a myriad of other benefits when it comes to **extending your life** as well. A fitter body is one that runs more efficiently. Your blood pressure is reduced and your risk factors for disease come down as well. You will find that all your internal systems work better when you are fitter – this has the knock-on benefit of making your body more easily able to fight signs of disease and aging and more easily able to maintain a healthy weight.

In fact, exercise can be so effective that it can help to completely reverse lifestyle diseases such as insulin resistance and diabetes. Jogging is such an effective form of exercise because it really is easy, in expensive and can match all levels of fitness. You can progress at your own pace – choose to join a club or use the time jogging as your own personal alone time, it just depends on what suits you best. Jogging on a treadmill allows you to completely zone out and forget about daily stresses. Jogging outdoors allows you to commune with nature and also forget about daily stresses.

In both instances, you will find that your blood pressure and other bodily functions become better regulated.

Use Exercise to Stress Less

Exercise helps to keep our bodies in better shape but has other benefits as well. Regular exercise helps to dissipate cortisol in the bloodstream and helps us to relax – combating the negative impact of stress. This is extremely important in terms of longevity. Prolonged stress and exposure to cortisol increases the amount of inflammation in the body and suppresses your immune response. You are more likely to pick up all bugs going around and are also less likely to be able to heal yourself as quickly.

Stress causes the deterioration of cells in the body and brain and so contributes to the deterioration associated with aging.

Better Circulation and a Better Body

Exercise helps to improve the circulation of the body both in terms of blood and lymph drainage – it thus helps to oxygenate the body and helps to speed the removal of toxins. This, in turn, helps with the turnover rate of the skin – you feel and look younger. Exercise helps to improve the shape of the body and will help you to lose weight.

Exercise to Fight Disease

The number one mass murderer of our day is the "silent killer" – heart disease. The number one tool in the fight against heart disease is cardiovascular exercise. Jogging is a great way to get yourself fitter without placing too much strain on the heart. It can be an invaluable tool in the fight against insulin resistance by helping to regulate hormone levels and the levels of sugar in the bloodstream. Insulin resistance, if left unchecked, will eventually progress to Type II Diabetes – the second biggest killer in this day and age.

Jogging for Better Bones

Women are at particular risk for developing osteoporosis as they age. Getting enough calcium in your diet will only get you so far in the quest for stronger bones. Weight bearing exercise, like jogging, where stress is placed on the bones, gets you the rest of the way.

How to Get into Jogging

It is pretty easy to start jogging – all you need to do is to get a comfortable pair of sneakers that provide the right support for your feet. From there it is just a matter of deciding where you will jog. Here it does help if you have an exercise buddy to motivate you. Again, as with any exercise program, start off slowly at a level that matches your current fitness level. If you haven't exercised in a while or are very unfit, consider walking at a brisk pace for about two or three minutes and then jogging for one minute.

Change it up like this throughout your workout. As you get fitter, you can increase the amount of time you spend jogging. Eventually, when you are able to jog for the whole time, you can intersperse the jogging with sprinting to further increase your fitness levels. Interval training in this way has been proven to be a more effective tool for overall fitness and is a great way to maximize the benefits of exercising overall.

ACTION PLAN

- Check whether or not there is a jogging club in your area – jogging can be quite a social experience.

- Get yourself a comfortable pair of sneakers. You do not need to get the most expensive brand but do look for good quality shoes.

- If you will be jogging through your neighborhood, take a drive around your proposed route in your car, taking note of the starting and ending speedometer readings. Now you know the exact distance of your route.

- If you have an MP3 player, set up a killer music routine that energizes you and pumps you up.

- Find a suitable stretching routine so that you will properly warm your muscles before setting out.

- Set up goals for yourself now that you know how long your proposed route is. Make deals with yourself – start off by jogging to the corner and seeing how you do – you may be surprised by how much you can actually do. Maybe set the next corner as the next goal, etc.

Everyday Habit #107

NEVER Forget This

Always get your daily fruit and vegetable intake daily - Every single day, seven days a week, 365 days a year. This is one of the single most helpful health tips and one that is easy to implement. It is also one that a lot of us fail at. Very few people in the Western world eat the full 5-9 servings of fruit and vegetables a day and we are feeling the consequences in terms of lifestyle diseases.

Obesity has become a global epidemic and every year, millions of new cases of cardiovascular disease and Type II Diabetes are diagnosed. These are the two biggest killers of our time and the sad thing is that following a healthy diet and getting enough exercise can easily prevent these diseases. The typical western diet leaves the body starving for nutrients and fiber because it revolves around highly refined carbohydrates and unhealthy fats.

The Refined Carb Crises

Never before have we had so much access to such a wide variety of food, or food that is so refined. The problem with eating a lot of refined carbs is that they are non-nutritive but extremely addictive. You may as well mainline sugar; refined carbs have a similar effect on the body. The more you eat, the more you want to eat. Fortunately, you can wean yourself off these dreadful "foods".

Need some encouragement to break the carb habit? Getting enough fruit and vegetables on a daily basis can reduce the chances of developing **heart disease** by as much as 76% and can also reduce your chances of developing dread diseases such as **breast cancer**. The anti-oxidant value of nature's power foods can also reduce the risks of developing cancer and help your body to fight the signs of aging – they are the best anti-wrinkle treatments available today.

Your waistline will also benefit simply by increasing the amount of vegetables and fruit that you eat. The fiber in them helps to make your digestive system work more smoothly and helps to keep you feeling fuller. The low-calorie density means that you are less likely to gain weight if these are included in your diet.

Fruit and veggies contain a large proportion of water – eating enough of these foods raw can contribute significantly to the proper hydration of your entire body. Fruit and veggies are Mother Nature's fast foods – most of them are highly portable and can be eaten with hardly any processing or preparation. Reaching for a carrot rather than a chocolate bar does not come naturally but, if you think about it, both are equally easy to use as snacks.

It's A Lot Easier Than You Think

Getting the recommended amount of fruits and vegetables is a lot easier than you think. You should aim to eat around about 2 ½ cups of vegetables a day and about 3 or 4 servings of fruit. This is quite easy – a small apple by itself is one serving of fruit, so adding an apple to each meal means that you will automatically get the right amount of fruit every day. You shouldn't just stop at apples though – eating a variety of fruit and veggies ensures that you get range of different nutrients. The more varied your diet, the more nutrients you are going to get. You want your diet to be as colorful as possible. Carrots, for example, are rich in beta-carotenes. Blueberries are high in anti-oxidants.

Eat Them Raw and Wriggling

Okay, so Gollum's advice from the Lord of the Rings movie pertains to rabbits or fish but it is good advice when it comes to fruit and vegetables as well – you want to get them as fresh as possible and prepare them as little as possible. The more they are processed, the more nutrients that are lost. Ideally, all you should need to do is to wash them carefully and, if possible, eat the fruit or veggie and peel as well.

How to Wash Fruit and Veggies

If you cannot source organic produce or cannot grow it yourself, it is important to wash away any residue that may be on the produce. Add a half a cup of vinegar to a sink full of water and soak produce in that for at least 10 minutes to get rid of residues. If the vinegar idea does not appeal to you, simply soaking the produce in plain water will also help. Scrub before serving to ensure that it is really clean.

To Peel or Not to Peel, that is the Question

Most fruit and vegetable peels are edible. It is important to make use of this valuable resource as the peels usually contain more fiber and nutrients than the flesh of the plant. This is where growing your own veggies can be invaluable. For pretty much my whole life, I thought that the peels of the gem squash were inedible. When I started growing my own, I found out that the skin is actually a lot softer just after you have picked the gem squash and that you can actually cook and eat it in stews, etc. It is as the squash ages off the vine that the skin becomes unpalatable and hard. The harder the skin, the longer the squash has been off the vine. Growing them yourself is the best way to ensure that no harmful pesticides are used in the process. And you do not always need a lot of space. Vertical veggie gardens and window boxes make it possible for the apartment dweller to have their own supply of fresh veggies – it is just a matter of finding the veggies suited to the space that you have.

Fresh is Best

Nothing beats the taste of a tomato that you have picked straight off the plant. Homegrown vegetables really do taste a whole lot better.

The bonus is that weeding, planting, etc. can be pretty good exercise as well. You also have no need to use pesticides, etc. – there are plenty of natural ways to deal with pests. You also know that your veggies are as fresh as possible when you grow them yourself. If you cannot grow them yourself, look out for a farmer's market in your area and see what you can get there. It is worthwhile getting there as the market opens so that you have your pick of what is on offer.

Modern life has done us a bit of a disservice in this regard – stores can now ship in produce from all over the world. This allows us to enjoy our favorite fruits and veggies year-round but was not what nature intended. It is better to stick to fruit that is currently in season – it will be less expensive and fresher – fruit that is flown in has been part of the cold chain much longer and was probably picked before properly ripe meaning that it is less flavorful anyway. It is also better to steer clear of the pre-cut fruit and vegetables. These are a lot more convenient but may have been treated with nasty chemicals to ensure that they don't go off quickly. Also, fruits and veggies start to deteriorate and lose nutrients once they have been sliced.

Frozen Can Work

If fresh is not a viable option, frozen is a good one. Most veggies and fruit are frozen shortly after being picked, locking the nutrients in. This does allow you to make use of a range of different vegetables and exotic fruits that may not grow in your area. The downside of frozen veggies is that they need to be cooked – they end up being a mushy mess otherwise. Cook them directly from frozen for the best results.

Get Sneaky

I started to grow my own veggies because I wasn't getting enough in my diet and I knew that home grown tasted better. Whenever I went home to my mom for a meal, she would get sneaky and toss in some veggies. For example, if she made chicken mayo sandwiches, she would add grated carrot – you didn't really taste the carrot but it was there. Think of sneaky ways to add fruit and veggies if you really don't like the flavor of them. Grating veggies is a great way to avoid chunks of veggies in meat dishes and stews – you can sneak grated veggies in a lot more easily than diced ones. Once again, I'll use the example of grated carrots – they can make a meatloaf much more nutritious and help it be moister at the same time.

Find New Ways to Prepare Veggies

Personally, I'm not a fan of cauliflower or carrots. Chop them up as crudités and serve with hummus and I'll eat lots of them. Another favorite of mine is grated carrot with chunks of fresh pineapple and a bit of pineapple juice. What I am getting with here is that you need to experiment with ways to prepare you fruit and veggies so that they taste good and you enjoy eating them. That way, it is easy to get the minimum amounts.

Smoothies Can Help

Another way that I incorporate veggies is with smoothies. I add in my favorite fruits, a banana, some milk, some almonds and then the veggies that I know I should be eating but wouldn't touch otherwise, like celery. I'll often throw in some wheatgrass or carrots as well. The smoothie tastes great and gives me a great energy boost.

Cut the Juice

Fruit and vegetable juices, on the other hand, are a bad idea. Even if you make your own juices at home, you are losing out on a lot of valuable fiber.

Without this fiber, the natural sugar content in the juices can cause havoc in your system. Fruit and veggies are designed to be eaten with their fiber, not without it.

Consider Replacing the Fat with Fruit

If you are baking, you can often substitute a good portion of the fat for applesauce, as one example, with little impact in terms of results and flavor. This can be a great way to allow you to still enjoy baked goods that are healthier and lighter and better for you.

ACTION PLAN

- List the fruit and vegetables that you enjoy and put them on your shopping list – even if it means getting frozen varieties.

- Find out about upcoming farmer's markets in the area and plan your day accordingly. Farmer's markets can be a fun event – you can often find great deals, meet up with friends and get a nice healthy breakfast to boot.

- See if there are family-run farms in the area that will supply produce. What some farmers do is to send out a box of whatever fruit and vegetables look best for that week – you get a fresh supply and variety quite easily.

- Start looking for new recipes that incorporate fresh produce.

- If you do establish a veggie garden, you can swop excess produce with other home gardeners to get an even bigger variety.

Everyday Habit #108

Cut Out The CRAP!

We know that junk food is bad for us. We know that excessive drinking is bad for us. We know that smoking is bad for us. Why then, do we carry on punishing our bodies? It is probably because doing the right thing can initially be uncomfortable. Having that drink or smoke feels good at the time and, let's face it, a cheeseburger tastes a lot better than a salad most of the time. We tend to go for the path of least resistance – the easy way out, not realizing how ill we actually are. Speak to someone who has stopped smoking or started to follow a healthy eating plan and what do they have in common? They will generally tell you that they feel better than they have in years – with more energy and vitality.

I believe that the main problem is that we become used to feeling less than our best – we are free of "serious" illness but do not feel well either. Life takes its toll and we forget what real health is like. It has become natural to "feel your age". After all, aging is inevitable, isn't it? Except that it really is not. Aging is not really a natural phenomenon – think about it, how many of our distant ancestors actually made it to old age before becoming some animal's dinner or falling victim to some illness? The fact that some people age well and others become so frail is testament to the fact that aging is more a sign of wear and tear than a natural progression. This is great - it means that there is a lot that we can do about it. Living right is your key to success. You know what I am going to say next, don't you? Living right does not include smoking, excessive drinking or junk food.

Right about now, most people will have some story about someone that they knew that smoked a pack of cigarettes a day until they were in their seventies.

My own grandmother smoked 30 a day and lived until she was 74. But then, the stresses and strains she had in her life were very different. She also made sure that we all ate our fruit and veggies every day and had a cooked, healthy breakfast of oatmeal.

Combine any of the three under-mentioned vices and you have a winning combination – if your aim is to cash out early. I keep thinking that my own grandmother would have lived longer if she had not smoked. Her best friend, who grew up on a neighboring farm, never smoked a day in her life and carried on till the ripe old age of 91. I can't help feeling that I got short-changed. My grandma should have been around a lot longer. If you want to be there for your grandkids or if you are serious about living to be 100 and still being vital at that age, you need to cut out the crap. Make that decision right now and start right now.

Smoking

You know all those articles about how smoking is good for you? They do not exist. You know that it is bad for you. You know that you'll be better off without it. I don't have to go into all the reasons why. You know what they are and you are probably sick of hearing them. You probably have some quick comebacks to justify smoking. Not one of them is good enough. You are not going to quit smoking tomorrow – if you are serious about your health, quit this instant. Make the decision now and you will be a lot healthier for it.

Alcohol

My ex used to say that he had no problem drinking and he was right. His problem was stopping. Once he had one drink, he just carried on drinking until he passed out. The occasional glass of red wine can be good for you – it has a high anti-oxidant content and can help you to relax but don't kid yourself, there are much better sources of antioxidants. If you need alcohol to relax or you can't stop at just one glass of wine, you have a problem and you need to start dealing with it.

Alcohol, if consumed to excess over a long period of time will damage your internal organs and make you seem to age a lot faster. You could have the liver of a fifty-year-old at the ripe old age of 30. It will also cut your lifespan. It just isn't worth it.

Junk Food and Sugar

You may not realize this but junk food and sugar can rate as dangerous as alcohol and cigarettes if consumed in excess. In fact, they can be even more dangerous – no one is going to moan at you if you eat two cheeseburgers but they may complain if you have two bottles of wine. While there is a serious social backlash against smokers – simply lighting up is likely to make people look at you as they would a serial killer – there is not nearly the same amount of outrage for someone who overdoes the junk food.

In fact, most people will look at you with some degree of pity if you are obese – or think that you have no willpower. They are not likely to come right out and tell you that you are slowly killing yourself. Eating junk food is a lot more sociably acceptable than lighting up but just as dangerous. Junk food and sugar act on the same pleasure centers in the brain that drugs act on. We get a bit of a buzz from eating sugar and junk food. That is why they taste so good and why it is so hard to cut them out completely. Sugar addiction is becoming more recognized as a valid eating disorder, viewed along the same lines as bulimia and anorexia. There are support groups out there for people who are addicted to junk food.

What you need to understand is that you need support to help kick the sugar habit, just like any other addict does. This is not a harmless addiction either. The problem with junk food is that it provides empty calories, and lots of them. You could eat junk food all day, every day and still be regarded as undernourished. Junk food is usually so refined that most of the nutrients are long gone. It is pumped full of sugar and then usually deep-fried. It may taste great but that cheeseburger can be deadly if you eat too many of them. The trans-fats in the foods cause inflammation in your body and this, in turn, damages the cardiovascular system and can lead to the development of heart disease. Science is now finding that overconsumption of sugar is one of the leading causes of diseases today. Eating too much sugar leads to spikes in the blood sugar levels and the storage of fat in the liver and around your abdominal organs.

Eventually, your body becomes resistant to insulin and you gain even more weight and so a vicious cycle begins that is tough to break. I am not saying that you can never have another cheeseburger, just that you have to be limiting the number of cheeseburgers that you eat. Aim to eat a healthy diet at least 80% of the time and you should be okay. The only cautionary note here is that this only works if you can control your intake of junk food. If eating one bit of junk food is going to send you into binge mode, it is not worth taking the risk.

Like any other addiction, once you do break the junk food habit, you will find it easier to eat healthy foods again. It takes just two weeks of having no sugar at all to completely break the sugar habit – after that, you are free and clear of the cravings.

ACTION PLAN

- If you smoke, quit now. Planning so that you are "ready" to quit is just one way of delaying quitting. Whether you quit today or tomorrow, it is going to be tough. Get started today and you will already be one day closer to being able to go without a cigarette.

- How much do you drink? One glass of wine with supper is not such a bid deal. Do you stop there though? Or do you save up all your units for a weekend binge?

  If you feel that you may have a bit of a problem, even if it is not so bad, seek support in the form of an AA class to prevent it progressing.

- Check your cupboards. How many sugary items do you have in them? What about junk food? Check the labels of items in your cupboard. If sugar tops the list of items, or is in the top 3-5 ingredients, toss that out.

- Start reducing the amount of sugar you add to your food and drinks now. Your body learns to like sweet things, it can learn to unlike them again. Don't bother adding artificial sweeteners; just reduce the amount of sugar in your diet to a minimum.

- Keep yourself clear of temptation – don't buy the offending foods or drinks – if they are not easily accessible, it will be easier to resist them.

- You can give yourself a break once in a while when it comes to junk food, as long as it is not often. Schedule one day a week when you can have junk food for supper. Steer clear of it the rest of the time.

- Keep healthy alternatives. Most of the time, reaching for a packet of crisps is more a matter of habit than anything else. Keep healthy snacks on hand to help out at these times.

- Never go shopping when hungry.

- Think of something that you can do in place of drinking/ smoking/ eating junk food. Something that helps to take your mind off what you are "missing" out on.

Everyday Habit #109

Reduce Sun Time

We all need a little sunshine in our lives –Studies have shown that not getting enough exposure to daylight can lead to conditions like seasonal affect disorder. That said, around about 15 minutes of daily exposure to the sun, unprotected, in order to keep our Vitamin D levels up, is really all you need to stave off problems. Anything more than that is not only excessive but can be extremely damaging. Lying in the sun for hours is essentially the same as slow-roasting your skin. A tan is basically your skin's defense mechanism against exposure to UV radiation.

Despite the fact that we are a generation that worships tanned and toned bodies, spending time in the sun can really damage the skin, making it age faster and setting you up to develop skin cancer. The days of sun worshipping are over. If you really want that tanned look, it is much safer to get it out of a bottle – tanning beds are even worse for you than lying in the sun.

The fairer your skin, the more at risk you are of burning in the sun but fair people do have a bit of an advantage over their darker-skinned contemporaries – they know that staying out of the sun and wearing sunscreen is important. Darker skin can also burn and be damaged by the sun – no matter who you are, you need to wear the right sun protection. Sunscreen is the number one anti-aging cream on the market. There is nothing that can damage your skin as much as the sun can – it dehydrates the skin and breaks down the natural collagen leaving skin more prone to wrinkling and aging.

We All Scream for Sunscreen

Everyone, no matter what age they are, should be wearing sunscreen when venturing out of doors. The younger you start using sunscreen, the better your skin will look when you get older, so get your kiddies into the habit of using sunscreen now. You should apply a sunscreen of at least SPF 30 every time you go outside. That means before you leave for work, for lunch and before you go home.

And not only on your face – any area of skin that will be exposed to the sun should be covered. Your hands and neck are the areas of your body where signs of aging are most prevalent because these areas are usually exposed to the sun just as much as the face is but are usually afforded less protection.

Sun Wise Clothing

There are many clothing ranges that now also include UV protection in the fabric. Try and use these wherever possible. Shading yourself from the direct rays of the sun is also important – a wide-brimmed hat can be a face-saver. Long-sleeved tops, big sunglasses and long pants can also keep the sun off your skin. Choose lighter colors so that the rays bounce off and you feel cooler.

Careful Sun Exposure

Staying out of the sun when it is at its highest makes good sense – this is when it is at its strongest. That said, you need to watch out for reflected rays as well – even if you are sitting out of direct sunlight, the rays of the sun can cause damage if reflected onto you.

No Excuse to Skip the Sunscreen

Even if the day is overcast and miserable, you still need to put on sunscreen – radiation can penetrate the cloud layer and cause damage to the skin.

ACTION PLAN

- Go and buy a sunscreen with an SPF of at least 30 now.
- Use it every day – do not forget areas like the tips of your ears and scalp.
- Buy yourself a decent pair of sunglasses with a proper SPF to protect your eyesight – paying a bit more here is worthwhile.
- Get a big sunhat or cap to protect your face and neck from the sun.
- Monitor how much sun exposure you are getting overall.

Everyday Habit #110

The MOST Important Drink

Considering that your body is made up of almost 70% water, it should not surprise you that water is the MOST important drink of all. Water is used by every organ and system in the body, even being mildly dehydrated interferes with the smooth operation of the body.

Without water, you would not be able to regulate your body temperature, be as mobile or even oxygenate all the cells of the body. Without water, we die. It is that simple.

Fortunately, keeping yourself hydrated is really simple – you just need to drink more water. It's cheap, it's easy and it is a great anti-aging treatment. There is no moisturizer or face cream in the world that can compare to the proper hydration of the skin from the inside out.

8 Glasses a Day

Most health and wellness magazines suggest drinking 8 glasses of water a day in order to be properly hydrated. The truth is that even this may not be enough. The bigger your body, the more water you need. That said, you don't have to go and try and work out complicated formulas relating to your body mass and the amount of water to drink. Your body is really smart – drink water as soon as you feel thirsty. Just keep a bottle of the life-giving stuff to hand so that you can sip as required.

The great news is that it is easy to acquire a taste for water – drink it plain or with ice and in a few weeks, you will be looking forward to your daily water. Eventually, you will be able to taste the difference between water from different areas. If you really do not like the taste of plain water, add in some slices of fruit or some mint or cucumber to flavor it naturally. It is better to avoid the commercially available flavored waters as most contain a lot of sugar.

Get into the habit of having a glass of water with each snack and meal and you will automatically be drinking 3-5 glasses of water a day. You'll soon notice a difference in your skin – your skin will look clearer and more radiant. Getting enough water can also have significant benefits when it comes to your urinary tract – you will find that you are less prone to urinary tract infections. You will also find that you tend to eat less – many times what we interpret as hunger pangs is actually thirst. Drink a glass of water next time you feel as though you are hungry and see if that feeling goes away.

Does it Have to Be Bottled Water?

Whether you drink tap or bottled water will largely depend on the water quality in your area. There have been many cases where it has been found that bottled water has simply been taken from taps anyway. Mineral water can contain higher levels of minerals such as calcium, etc. than what you need. Tap water will usually contain chemicals to purify it. Having a filtration system fitted to your home taps is a good compromise between the two.

ACTION PLAN

- Get yourself a glass bottle that can hold at least 500ml of water. Glass is better because it keeps the water at a more even temperature and there is less chance of chemicals leaching into the water.

- Have the bottle on hand and drink from it whenever you feel thirsty or when you remember – thirst is a sign that dehydration has begun so you should try to aim to minimize thirst.

- Replace your daily soda with a glass of ice-cold water flavored with mint and cucumber. It is a lot more refreshing and healthy for you.

Everyday Habit #111

Floss Daily

This could be essential if you want to keep your arteries in good shape. Confused? Your mouth has nothing to do with your arteries, right? Wrong! The bacteria present in the mouth that can cause gum disease can enter the bloodstream and cause inflammation of the arteries. Inflammation of the arteries is what drives heart disease so keeping your mouth healthy can keep your heart healthy as well.

The **New York University** conducted a study in 2008 that concluded that daily flossing was necessary in order to reduce the amount of these bacteria overall. Further research has shown a link between higher levels of gum-disease causing bacteria and higher levels of arterial thickening. One expert recommends flossing twice daily in order to get the best benefits in terms of the extension of your life expectancy.

Isn't Brushing Enough?

Unfortunately, brushing is not enough – there are too many crevices between the teeth that your standard toothbrush is unable to reach. If you don't floss, food debris builds up in these areas and decays, providing the perfect breeding ground for bacteria. This causes bad breath and can end up damaging the enamel of the teeth.

Over time, you will develop gingivitis and if this is left unchecked, the infection can spread to the bone – from which point it is extremely painful and difficult to treat.

Plaque Makes You Look Older

The buildup of plaque on the teeth can cause discoloration that can make you look older than you really are. Our teeth get naturally duller and more stained as we age but this effect can be reduced if you look after your teeth well. And that means brushing and flossing need to be considered not only as part of your daily health routine but also as part of your daily beauty routine.

Visit Your Dentist

Your dentist can advise you on how to floss and pinpoint areas that you may not be reaching. Going every 6 months makes it possible to pinpoint problems early on and will mean that hard tartar buildup is regularly removed. In addition to flossing, there are other tricks that you can use to reduce the amount of bacteria in the mouth.

Eat Less Sugar

The bacteria in the mouth thrive on sugar. Eating less sugar overall will help in the battle to keep these bacteria in check. Always rinse your mouth out with plain water after eating anything sweet to lessen the impact on the teeth.

Consider Xylitol

Xylitol has been clinically proven to starve the bacteria responsible for gum disease. The bacteria absorb the xylitol but cannot digest it. They are then unable to digest the nutrients that they need and thus starve. For this tactic to be effective, you need to expose your teeth to xylitol at least 5 times a day. Chewing sugar-free gum that contains xylitol can help to keep your breath fresh and also to clear out the harmful bacteria in your mouth.

Eat More Raw Crunchy Fruits and Veggies

Not only are these naturally lower in sugar, but they also provide friction against the teeth and help to naturally reduce the incidence of plaque formations.

Rinse Your Mouth after Every Drink or Meal

It is best to rinse your mouth with plain water after every meal or drink so that you can help to prevent the buildup of plaque and bacteria. It is important to use plain water with no additives. Keeping a toothbrush on hand and dry-brushing (without toothpaste) after lunch or a snack can also help.

ACTION PLAN

- Get some dental floss today and learn how to use it.

- If you find it hard to use traditional floss, you can find dental picks and other tools that make flossing a lot easier. Many of these tools have the required amount of dental floss stretched and ready for use. You simply clean between your teeth – it is easy and simple.
- Keep a spare toothbrush in your desk for dry-brushing. (Get one of those anti-bacterial caps so that it doesn't pick up nasty bacteria).
- Keep toothpicks on hand to help remove larger particles of food when you cannot get to the floss.

Everyday Habit #112

Breakfast Really is the MOST Important Meal

Breakfast is not considered the most important meal of the day for nothing. Research has consistently found that those who have a healthy breakfast in the morning are less likely to be overweight and overeat for the rest of the day. People who eat breakfast have been reported to feel better both in terms of their mental and physical health. The verdict is in – breakfast is an important way to start your day. According to the Mayo Clinic, a mix of carbohydrates, protein and a little fat makes for a perfectly balanced breakfast. Another key is to ensure that you mix the breakfast up a little from day to day so that you get the right balance of nutrients.

Breakfast Boosts Metabolism

A good breakfast in the morning will boost your metabolism early in the day. You can thus rev up the amount of fat you burn from earlier on than would be the case if you skipped breakfast altogether.

Less Overall Calories

People who eat breakfast have been found to consume fewer calories overall than those who do not. In fact, those who skip breakfast are more likely to reach for the high calorie snacks than those who do not. So, the myth that some dieters seem to cling to – that eating breakfast only makes you hungrier – does definitely not hold true.

The Key with Breakfast

When it comes to breakfast, the key is to eat a good breakfast – with slow release carbs, lean protein, vegetables of some sort and some healthy fat. I will go into greater detail on what constitutes a good breakfast in the next chapter.

ACTION PLAN

- Examine why you do not eat breakfast – is it because you are constantly rushing out the door? If so, start waking up earlier so that you have time to eat breakfast.

- Is it because you don't feel hungry in the morning? You can easily get into the habit of eating breakfast, even if you are not that hungry – just choose food that you can stomach.

- If you do eat breakfast, what does it consist of? Does it meet the minimum requirements as laid out by the Mayo Clinic?

Everyday Habit #113

The RIGHT Breakfast

Eating the right breakfast every day is the key to success. According to a study conducted by Ferrucci and his associates, a serving of whole-grains, especially when eaten in the morning seems to help people on the older side to have steadier levels of blood sugar all through the day. The study found that those who include a serving of whole grains in the morning also have a lower risk of developing diabetes – known to accelerate the aging process. It is thought that the high fiber content of these breakfasts is what helps with the supply of steady levels of blood sugar.

The ideal is to eat between 25g-35g of fiber every day. If you have been following a low fiber diet up until this stage, it is better to add increase your fiber intake more slowly as this will reduce the side effects. Increased amounts of fiber can lead to increased flatulence and stomach cramps, especially when the amount of fiber taken in is increased quickly.

Great Carbs for Breakfast

There has been a lot of press about the value of a low-carb diet with those supporting this eating plan and those who are against it completely. The trick when eating carbs is in keeping them complex. That way, they provide a steady flow of energy without spiking your blood sugar levels.

Oats are a great source of carbohydrates, as long as you stick to traditional oats and steer clear of the traditional kind. Serve with a little fresh butter, some sliced fruit and a tub of yoghurt on the side and you have a perfect breakfast. Oat bran is another simple breakfast food that can be easily used to increase the amount of fiber in your diet. Serve over oats or eat on its own for a daily dose of fiber. Mixed with warm milk and a little cinnamon, it is quite tasty.

One caution here – be careful to check the ingredients of any wholegrain cereals that you are considering buying. Take granola, for example, it may seem to be healthy but usually contains a lot of sugar. Even so-called healthy all-bran cereals can be laced with sugar to make them taste better. You can also get quite creative with breakfasts – there is nothing that says that breakfast has to be boring. What about adding in some Quinoa – either as an omelet filling or as porridge? Polenta makes a great, filling grain, as does millet. Use your imagination – the less processed the grain, the less likely it will be to spike your blood sugar.

Protein is Essential

Protein should be eaten at each meal. Protein helps to stabilize blood sugar and quell hunger pangs. It is an essential nutrient to keep your body younger and stronger. You don't even need to have much of it – one egg, a small tub of yoghurt or a piece of salmon the same size of your palm are all good examples of proteins that you can add to your daily diet.

If you do choose yoghurt, it is important to stick to Greek yoghurt that is sugar-free. You can add a little honey to sweeten it if you want to but normally it is enough just to add in some fresh fruit for a bit of sweetness. Commercial low-fat yoghurts should be eaten infrequently or not at all. They are packed with sugar. When it comes to the protein that you choose, try to source it from suppliers who raise the animals naturally – grass-fed beef, free-range chickens, etc. The nutritional value of such food is a lot higher.

Just a Little Bit of Fat

We have all been taught that fat is bad but the latest research has turned this on its head. Scientists now advise that you need to get about 35% of your calories from fat. It turns out that some fat is actually good for you! That means no more having to fry your eggs in a little water – you can use butter if you want to. This is great news. Fat is a very tasty and satisfying food – it can also help to slow the release of sugar into the bloodstream.

This does not mean that you can go overboard – about a tablespoon of olive oil/ butter or peanut butter counts as one serving of fat. If you are not keen on oils, you can add nuts or seeds instead – half an ounce counts as one serving in this case.

Get Your Fruit/Veggie Serving

It may seem weird to talk about adding veggies to your breakfast but there are lots of ways to do this naturally. You could make a veggie-filled omelet or a frittata, for example. Even fried tomato or mushrooms on the side of the plate do count. Ideally, you should look at about half a plate full of veggies at breakfast to really rev up your veggie intake. You can get quite creative with them – why not have roasted veggies instead of boiled ones? Put a little butter over them for extra flavor and they'll taste great.

Most people are accustomed to having fruit with their breakfast. It's a great way to add a bit of sweetness and flavor without overdoing the sugar content. When it comes to stable blood sugar, fruits with high sugar content like bananas are best kept to a minimum. Apples are in the mid-GI range and berries come out in the low-GI range. Once again, mixing it up a bit every day will ensure that you get a great range of nutrients.

ACTION PLAN

- What cereals, etc. do you have in your cupboards at the moment? Get rid of the unhealthy ones.

- Go out and get a bag of oats – they are a very versatile standby for breakfast. If you want a quick fix for breakfast, they can be eaten raw. Alternatively, soak them overnight in water or milk and heat in the morning for a quick and tasty breakfast.

- Make a list of whole grains that you would like to try and find out how to prepare them.

- Considering preparing extra grains at suppertime for use the next morning.

- Gather some recipes – there are stacks on the Internet – to make breakfast more interesting. What about Polenta cakes and salmon, for example?

Everyday Habit #114

Eat Food, Not Supplements

Research has shown that people who have higher levels of some nutrients in their blood, such as beta-carotene, selenium and Vitamins C and E, for example, tend to be healthier for longer as they age. This has resulted in the supplement industry putting forth many anti-aging compounds and these appear to have been well-adopted as well.

We all seem to be willing to try short-cuts when it comes to our health. The problem is that there is no scientific evidence that taking these elements as a supplement actually contributes to anti-aging. When it comes to nutrition, we simply have to bow to Mother Nature – she is a master-chemist. Take the humble tomato, for example, this can contain as many as 200 separate flavonoid compounds and 200 separate carotenoid compounds in just one piece of fruit. According to Ferrucci, the interaction between these various chemicals is a lot more important when it comes to wellbeing than the chemical breakdown as a whole.

In nature, the various chemicals work together to support one another. Our science is not yet advanced enough to replicate this interaction. What this boils down to is that there are no real shortcuts when it comes to health. You need to fuel your body with real food that contains valuable nutrients if you want to be as healthy as possible. And keeping the food as near as possible to its natural state enables you to get the best benefits. The more processed the food is, the less nutrients it contains.

Eating simple, fresh and healthy food is the best way to keep your body looking and feeling younger for much longer. You can take a basic multi-vitamin supplement to ensure that there are no deficiencies in your diet but you cannot rely on supplements alone to ensure that you get the right nutrition.

Eating a wide range of real food is the only way to make sure that your body gets all the nutrients that it needs and can use.

ACTION PLAN

- How much real food do you eat?

- How much processed food do you have in your cupboards? That's right, it's time to clear it out.

- Start adding more whole foods to your grocery list.

- Look online for easy recipes that making cooking these whole foods a lot more convenient.

- When cooking, cook double quantities and save half for another meal. Let the food cool completely before putting it into freezer bags/ containers. Be sure to label carefully with the date made and what the meal is before you put it in the freezer.

Everyday Habit #115

Go with The Flow

We all know at least one person who is completely neurotic – isn't it amazing how often things tend to go wrong for them? Doesn't it seem like anything that can go wrong does go wrong? Think about the words that you use to describe the neurotic people in your life – drama queen – is that a title that you hold? Or is it one to aspire to?

The truth is that everyone has his or her problems and no one wants to be around a drama queen all the time. Think about someone you know that fits the bill. How seriously do you take them? Aren't you prone to think that they are over-exaggerating all the time? If you are the drama queen, ever notice how people just do not seem to take you as seriously anymore? Wood Allen seems to make neurosis look cool and funny but the reality is that it is not the best way to go through life, especially not if you want to live to be a hundred.

In studies of centenarians, one common thread was the way that they dealt with stress and problems – they tended to be very resilient and didn't let life get them down too much. They had learned to go with the flow and tended to have better support structures in place than the constant worriers.

If you are a natural born worrier, this can be a trait that is difficult to unlearn but there are ways to do this. Finding a healthy outlet for your stress and learning how to relax will help improve both your quality of life and longevity.

Does it Really Matter?

Don't believe me? The next time you are worried about something, think about whether or not it will matter in a year's time, or 5 years' time. There are very few worries that actually do stand the test of time – most of the time we are just wasting energy worrying about some imagined slight or some issue that really isn't worth five minutes thought, let alone the hours and hours that we are spending on it.

The bad news is that the more you think about a problem, the more important it becomes in your mind and the more that you will want to think about it. Misery loves company – one worrying idea is being bound to lead to another and pretty soon you will have an entire doomsday scenario worked out in your mind. And the more time you give the idea, the more you will want to think about it.

The Elephant in the Room

Take an elephant, for example. Right now, I bet you are picturing an elephant. What does that elephant have to do with this conversation? Absolutely nothing but I'll bet you are still picturing that elephant. See how that works? Because I was constantly bringing up the elephant, even though it had no bearing on the situation, you thought of it. Right, now stop thinking about the elephant. Not that simple, is it? Simply telling yourself not to think about it is not a good coping strategy. You need to find a way to really put it out of your mind.

Worries can take over your mind in a very similar way, even if they have little or no bearing on your current situation. Your boss was probably a little short with you today because they had something else on their mind. They are probably not avoiding you because they want to fire you. You are not likely to miss the mortgage payment and have your house repossessed. The chances are not that good that you will end up on the street. In fact, the reason that your boss was short with you probably has a lot less to do with you than you think but we tend to be wired to think that we are the center of our universe – we think that everything revolves around us.

The truth is that your boss probably feels that they are the center of their own universe too – they probably didn't even realize that they slighted you.

Find out How to Cope

You need to learn some real coping skills and relaxation techniques. One technique that can be very effective is to have a worry session. You allow yourself to worry about a particular topic but set a timer on it – say 20 minutes. During your session, you are allowed to think of the direst outcomes that you can imagine, but when the timer goes, you have to get up and do something else to take your mind off worrying. If you have someone to talk to, that is great. Just be sure to keep the same limits in place and be sure that they understand that you don't need a sympathy session, you just want to get something off your chest.

Alternatively, it can be very useful to write down what is bothering you. Again, set a time limit on how long you will write for. The advantage of writing it down is that you get to get it off your chest and you can start to view it more objectively. Keep your "worry" diaries in a safe place and look over them in a few months' time – in most cases, you'll sit and laugh at what you were worried about at the time. This exercise is great to see what worries actually matter – very few do. This is where relaxation techniques and hobbies can come in very useful. Learning how to meditate or do yoga can be very relaxing. Not your scene? How about going for a walk or practicing your breathing?

Why not pull out your favorite movie – an uplifting one, or calling a friend for a quick chat? Sitting stewing for ages on the problem is not going to solve it – in fact, it can be downright counter-productive. Have you ever felt good after worrying for hours about something? How many of your worries actually materialized? If there is something that you can do about the situation, then do it. If there is nothing that you can do about it, then what is the point of worrying about it anyway? If you find that you simply cannot help yourself, it is a good idea to book a session with a psychologist – with the express purpose of learning better coping skills.

Considering the benefits in terms of health and wellbeing, learning to cope with the stresses and worries in your life is an excellent strategy. Sometimes all you need is to break that chain of thought. This is where it is useful to have a hobby that you can enjoy that engrosses you.

Throw yourself into your hobby when something is really bugging you – you'll break the chain of worry and get something productive and fun done instead. Isn't that a lot better than worrying about it?

ACTION PLAN

- Get your "worry" kit together now. Get a pad of paper or book to write in and make sure that you have a timer that works. If your worries are keeping you up at night, keep the notepad next to your bed and write them down. Often just committing them to paper can be enough to stop the worry cycle and let you sleep.

- Find self-help books on coping with stress and actually read them, or make an appointment to see a professional who can teach you coping techniques. Keep looking until you find techniques that work for you – not everything will work for everyone.

- Find something that you really enjoy doing – something that you can turn to in place of worrying, something that absorbs your attention fully so that you can break the worry chain.

- Learn relaxation techniques such as deep breathing and meditation and set aside time every day to practice these.

- Is there a friend that you can trust to speak to when you are worrying who will just listen without inciting you? Our friends do try to commiserate and show support but this can end up by making you feel more agitated rather than calming you down.

Everyday Habit #116

Build Habits

Like it or not, humans are creatures of habit. According to research by Olshasky, those who live to be a hundred tend to live lives governed by strict routine – they do not experience a lot of upheavals in their lives and tend to do the same thing and eat the same sort of things every day. This may seem boring but it does make sense as you get older. According to Ferrucci, your body becomes less resilient to change as you age.

Whereas in your twenties you may have been able to party until dawn and still worked a full day the next day, this will become impossible in your fifties. In fact, you may find that instead of being the life of the party, you become the party pooper. This is natural – even missing one night of sleep can have a serious effect on your physiology, especially as you get older – you simply cannot bounce back the way you did when you were younger and radical changes are more likely to have serious effects on your well-being and immune system, leaving you more open to contracting illnesses.

Something as simple as going to bed at the same time every night and waking up at the same time every morning can have dramatic effects in terms of health – your system settles into the routine and you find that you are well-rested and better able to cope with what life throws at you.

ACTION PLAN

- Start looking for ways to make life more routine. Start with your sleep/ wake cycle.

- Is there anything healthy that you can make a habit today? How about exercising first thing in the morning?

- Are there any habits that are better to break? Flopping down on the couch to vegetate in front of the TV as soon as you get home, for example.

Everyday Habit #117

Socialize

Humans are social creatures – regular social contacts with friends and loved ones make life better and not having someone to share your joys and pains with makes you more prone to depression and this can take years off your life. It is one of the reasons that so many elderly bereaved people often deteriorate so quickly when their loved ones have passed on. There are psychologists who believe that the biggest benefits of getting out of the house to exercise is that you usually get to socialize. Even if all you do is to walk to the store and back, you still benefit from daily interaction with other people.

Forming lasting relationships is also key as you get older – people who know you well will be able to tell if something is not quite right and will encourage you to go to the doctor – they will be able to pick up subtle differences that you may miss. This is especially important as you start to age. Having people whose opinions you trust is an important part of protecting yourself as you grow older. They will be able to let you know gently that something is amiss and you will know that you can trust them to do what is best for you. Forming lasting relationships does not come naturally to everyone but it is a skill that can be learned and it is one that needs to be fostered. The saying that "No man is an island" is particularly true in this day and age – we need someone to look out for us and someone who we can confide in.

By the same token, it is also nice to be a friend to other people as well – people need to feel loved, needed and wanted. Being there for your friends is just as importance to your own well-being as them being there for you. You do not need hordes of friends – only one or two really good ones are all that you really need. In fact, studies have shown that it is more valuable to have a handful of friends that know you really well and who you can connect with than to have a bunch of acquaintances that you really don't know all that well.

The societal ideal is a big bunch of friends that do everything together but the truth is that this is not normally the case – maintaining relationships is difficult, especially as individual members of the group grow and change. Making friends as an adult can be a little harder than it seemed to be as children but it is still possible. Many people are lonely and tend to end up stuck that way because they are afraid of making the first move. Fear of rejection holds a lot of people back from leading a richer and fuller life. Start by looking for people with similar interests to yours – joining a local club or church group is not new advice but it really does work. When meeting people for the first time, try to be more upbeat and ask questions about them – people love to talk about themselves and do not want to be around someone who moans about everything. Be a thoughtful person and be sincere and people will be drawn to you.

Once again, being sociable is a skill that can be learned and is one that is worth learning.

ACTION PLAN

- Start today by speaking to at least one new person every day – chat to someone in the line while you are waiting to pay for your groceries – most people will chat back and you may find that you get on well.

- Take time to ask people you interact with regularly how they are doing and make a point of remembering something personal about them as well.

  This can be as simple as finding out how their kids are doing – anything that demonstrates that you remember who they are and what you have spoken about before will make them feel as though they are important to you.

- People may not remember what you say to them but will remember how you make them feel. If you make someone feel good about themselves, they are more likely to want to spend more time with you. This can be a tricky one though – you need to pay them compliments that are sincere. People can usually see through someone who is faking it a mile away.

Everyday Habit #118

Cut Your TV Time

Face it – you probably spend too much time watching TV as it is. How many times have you binged by watching a TV series to the detriment of your gym time? Pushing the "Next" button on the remote is NOT exercise. In fact, TV can be downright dangerous for you. **An Australian study** of 8,800 adults with no history of heart disease found a correlation between the amount of time spent sitting in front of the TV and your risk of premature death and heart disease. Participants who watched four or more hours of TV per day were about 50% more likely to die from any cause than those who limited their TV consumption to less than two hours.

Still not convinced? **Researchers calculated** that each additional hour of TV watched means you're 11 percent more likely to die from any cause. No TV show is that great. Not even "Dancing with The Stars." With the range of TV shows and channels on offer, in combination with services like Amazon Prime, YouTube and Netflix, it has never been easier to get access to TV. It's not called the idiot box for nothing – watching TV is mindless entertainment. Granted, it is fun but it can really mess with problem solving skills – everything is handed to you on a silver platter – you don't need to sort things out for yourself like you do when reading, for example.

Think back to the last time a series that you enjoyed was cancelled. It annoyed you, didn't it – you wanted to see how it ended, didn't you? Logically speaking though, you should be able to imagine any ending that you wanted but I'll bet that you wanted to find out what happened next. The problem with being a couch potato is that you are a couch potato – you sit like a blob on the couch getting less exercise than you should and socializing less then you should – we've all done it, turned down a night on the town with our mates to stay in and watch the latest episode of our favorite show. Or just watching "one more episode" when you should really be going to bed and ending up sleeping late and skipping your morning exercise as a result.

You reach for the popcorn or junk food and enjoy your show rather than getting out there and enjoying life or doing something that is good for your body. Mindless snacking when watching TV is all too easy – how many times have you reached in to the packet only to realize that you have finished all the crisps or sweets without even really realizing that you were eating them? You simply munch away and pretty soon eating that snack in front of the TV becomes a habit that is tough to break. You start to associate watching TV with eating crisps, for example, and pretty soon you start craving crisps whenever you sit down to watch TV – whether you are hungry or not.

There is no question about it, TV makes us lazy – how many times have you watched some drivel on TV just because you were too lazy to get up and do something else? One of the famous comedians makes a joke of it – he says that when he was growing up, he was the remote but it really isn't that funny. Channel surfing can quickly become a habit and before you realize it, you are spending your whole evening in front of the TV, with nothing to show for it.

The problem is that it is the activity levels that suffer the most. It is a lot easier spending half an hour watching TV than spending that same time on the treadmill - guess which one is better for you overall. If you really have to get your daily fix of TV, try to exercise while watching. At least that way you still get some exercise in.

Otherwise, why not try something radical – instead of switching the TV on when you get home, leave it off for the evening and spend some quality time with your family? I never thought that I could live without my TV – I was addicted to my shows – I didn't watch soap operas but I found something to watch every night. Then one night the satellite dish got struck by lightning. Suddenly, there was no alternative – there was no TV to watch.

The repairman could only come the following week so I got used to not having a TV to watch – that week I found other things to occupy my time with. The satellite has been fixed now but I find that I barely switch the TV on anymore – I find that it is a waste of time. I also find that I now sleep better and have more energy as well and I don't feel that I am missing out on anything.

Experiment with going without TV for one day and then gradually increase that to one week. You might be surprised how you suddenly have time to do so much more and how your free time no longer seems to whizz past.

If you find that you cannot do without the TV, do yourself one favor at least – change channels manually. Getting up to change channels will mean that you do get some exercise, even if it is not much and will stop you channel surfing. Boredom might set in earlier and you may be more likely to switch off the TV. If all else fails, throw the batteries for the remote away.

There is always going to be another TV show to watch. You can never get the time wasted in front of the TV back though. Think of it this way – how much will it matter in a few years' time if you miss the latest episode of Game of Thrones?

Look at reruns of some of your favorite shows, as an example. They never really seem as good to you as you get older. I never used to miss a single episode of Star Trek growing up but now I find those same episodes quite boring.

ACTION PLAN

- Have a media blackout one night this week. No TV at all. Hide the remote if you have to.

- Cut back on the amount of TV you watch overall – start by taking back an hour a night. Once you start accounting for the time spent in front of the TV, you start to realize how much time is wasted on advertising, etc.

- Ration the amount of time you are allowed to watch TV and save this up for your favorite shows – no more marathons or endless reruns.

Everyday Habit #119

Eat Some Nuts Every Day

A handful of nuts a day will keep the doctor away. Nuts are one of nature's super foods and provide a very good alternative for those who want to get enough Omega-3s but who cannot handle the idea of taking a cod liver oil or fish oil supplement.

A Harvard study conducted over the course of 30 years found that those who ate nuts daily were 20% less likely to die from any cause throughout the course of the study than those who didn't. The **Harvard researchers** also found that the more often people had nuts, the lower their risk of death was. It is thought that this is down to the cholesterol-balancing qualities in the nuts and the range of nutrients in them.

Walnuts have the highest levels of Omega-3s so add these to your diet as a way to boost your levels of these essential fatty acids and in place of an Omega-3 supplement. As with anything, variety is the best way to get the best range of nutrients. Brazil nuts, for example, have high levels of Selenium. Almonds are rich in calcium. Varying the nuts that you eat will also prevent you from getting toxic amounts of nutrients. As mentioned before, Brazil nuts have high levels of Selenium in them – if you eat too many of them though, the Selenium rises to toxic levels in your body.

Most people avoid nuts because they are so calorie dense but this is actually a mistake – the fats in nuts are mainly monounsaturated making them a very healthy food to eat. Two tablespoons full makes for one serving so you don't even have to eat that many. If you are concerned that you may not be able to stop eating them once you start, divide the pack into individual serving sizes and only keep one or two servings on hand for the day.

Chop them up and add to your oatmeal or salads to give a satisfying crunch. Count them as a fat when adding to your diet in this manner. They are also a great source of protein and will give you a lot of energy. Keep a small packet of nuts in your desk drawer to give you an energy boost when needed. Normally speaking though, it is better to store nuts in the refrigerator – because of their high fat content it is possible for them to turn rancid easily. That is why you should also try to buy them as fresh as possible. Nut butters and milks can also make for nutritive and healthy dairy alternatives. Almond milk in particular is very nourishing, easy to make and very tasty.

Make your Own Almond Milk

Take one cup of nuts and add two parts water. Leave to soak overnight and then place in the blender. Add a teaspoon of vanilla essence for flavor. Strain out the almond meal and store in the refrigerator. Use within 2-3 days. The almond meal can be mixed in with your morning oatmeal for a great protein and nutrient boost. Use the milk in smoothies or in your coffee as an alternative to dairy or drink it on its own as an energy-giving alternative to coffee and sodas.

Alternatively, reserve the almond meal to use as a treatment for your skin. It can be used as a nourishing scrub – simply mix with enough water to form a paste and gently rub over skin. Leave in place for about 15 minutes before rinsing off. This is a great anti-aging and moisturizing treat for the face.

ACTION PLAN

- Find a bulk supplier of nuts – they are usually less expensive to buy in bulk. Buy a pound or two at a time so that you always have some on hand.

- Most stores that stock nuts also have seeds on offer – sunflower and pumpkin seeds make a great addition to nuts if you are looking to make a healthy snack pack. Round this off with coconut flakes for a real taste treat.

- It may be tempting to also add in dried fruit but keep this as an occasional treat rather than a daily one – dried fruit is a very concentrated source of sugar.

- It can be easier to figure out how many nuts form a portion instead of always having to measure quantities. Two tablespoons of almonds equals around about 14. Alternatively, fill an empty, clean yoghurt tub with the right amount and mark off the level on the tub. Cut the tub to match the marking and you will always get the portion size of nuts right.

- Nuts are healthy and good for you but can be fattening if eaten in excess. Eating handfuls at a time can seriously jeopardize your weight loss efforts.

Everyday Habit #120

Consume LESS Red Meat

Enjoying the odd burger or steak is not going to kill you but you do need to cut back on the red meat. **One study** found that women and men who were initially healthy had a higher chance of developing heart disease and cancer if they ate red meat on a regular basis. Having red meat everyday increases your chances of dying prematurely by 13%.

Processed meats, like lunchmeats and hot dogs are even worse and increase your chances of dying prematurely by 20%. Numerous studies have linked processed meats to higher incidences of cancer and cardiovascular disease.

It is not all doom and gloom though. I'm not advocating that you give up meat altogether – only that you cut back on the amount of red meat that you eat. Even if you have been eating red meats with abandon throughout your life, swapping these out for healthier proteins such as chicken and fish, or dairy products today can make a big difference.

Look for simple protein alternatives and get creative – you could find a whole new diet that gives you energy and is healthy for you as well. You don't have to stick to chicken and fish. Try something a little more exotic like ostrich meat – it is a high-quality protein that is very low in fat and very tasty.

Also consider adding in lentils, eggs, etc. There are a ton of great egg recipes out there. Eggs are one of the healthiest protein sources that we can get today – they are packed with nutrients and are very versatile. Cheeses can also substitute nicely for protein. The simple fact is that most of us overdo it in the meat department anyway. Take a look at the palm of your hand – one portion of meat is the size and thickness of your palm. Anything over and above that is too much.

How to Cook the Meat

It is also not just the type of meat that we eat but the way we cook it and how well we cook it that matters as well. There have been worrying studies that have linked grilled/ broiled and fried meat to an increased risk of developing cancer. One **study** showed that regularly eating burnt or charred meat (as many people do when enjoying barbequed meat) increases your chances of developing pancreatic cancer by as much as 60%.

Roasting meat is a better option overall – you just need to ensure that the internal temperature gets high enough to kill off potential pathogens. This is easily checked with a meat thermometer.

Cooking meat at high temperatures causes the formation of carcinogenic chemicals within the meat. Those that like their meat well-done are most at risk - This risk counts for all types of meat and not just for red meat.

Reduce the Risk

You can reduce the risk by cooking over lower temperatures. If you love your barbeques, trim off excess fat that can cause the fire to flare up and flip the meat regularly.

Marinating your meat can also go a long way towards reducing the potential for creating carcinogenic compounds during cooking. To get the full benefits, the meat should be marinated for at least half an hour but preferably overnight.

ACTION PLAN

- Start swapping out red meat for healthier meats such as fish and chicken.

- If you must eat red meat, have it no more than twice a week at the very most.

- Consider alternative sources of protein such as cheese and eggs.

- Look up new ways to prepare meat on the internet – ways that do not involve high heat cooking.

- Stock up on marinades and try to always marinade meat before cooking it – it improves the taste and the health value of the meal.

Everyday Habit #121

Eat More Sushi

Studies have found that Japanese women enjoy some of the **longest life spans** globally and it is thought that this is due to the food that they eat – traditionally, their diets contain a lot of sushi. Not only is the fish low in saturated fats but it is also high in Omega-3 fatty acids, known to reduce inflammation throughout the body. In a 2013 study, a diet high in consumption of Omega-3 fatty acids was linked to an overall **lower risk of dying** from all causes.

In order to get the right amount of Omega-3 fatty acids, you need to eat at least 2-3 servings of oily fish per week – what a great excuse to indulge your love of sushi? Because the fish is uncooked, there is no danger from the carcinogenic compounds formed during high heat cooking.

Get the Right Sauces with the Sushi

Traditional Wasabi paste can also have benefits in terms of health – it can boost metabolism and help to destroy the bacterium in the stomach that cause inflammation and cancer. You do need to check that the paste is made up from actual wasabi – "proper" wasabi is often mixed or replaced with horse radish. Whilst horse radish is also a good choice for health, wasabi is the better choice.

It can be almost impossible to taste the difference and it is important to check the labeling carefully as companies often color the horse radish green so that it looks like real wasabi. It helps to guard against food poisoning as well – good when you are eating raw fish. Most sushi is rolled in seaweed and this is one vegetable that packs a big punch in terms of nutrition. It has a number of minerals and vitamins in it so it is worth including in the diet. Paired with the sushi it hardly even tastes like a vegetable at all.

Overall, sushi is a winner when it comes to health and well-being. It is low in calories, high in nutrients and protein and a very satisfying meal. There are many different types of sushi making this one very versatile meal. The only caution here is to find a supplier or restaurant that works with the freshest fish. Sushi should not smell fishy or even taste overly fishy. If yours does, it is usually a sign that the fish is not as fresh as it should be.

You should also look at the flesh of the fish before eating it – it should have a pleasant tinge of color – if it is starting to go grey, it is probably not as fresh as it should be. If you are concerned about the freshness of the fish, it is better to skip it altogether – tainted fish can make you ill for days.

ACTION PLAN

- Find a good sushi restaurant near your home or office and treat yourself once a week. Some restaurants make a show of preparing the sushi and this can be quite interesting to watch.

- You should also consider learning how to make your own sushi. There are many kits available on the market and it is quite easy once you get the hang of it.

- If you have never tried sushi, get up the courage and go and try some – you never know, you may just love it.

Everyday Habit #122

Eat Chocolate!

Most of us, somewhere along the line, have made the argument that chocolate is actually a vegetable because it is derived from the cacao bean. Like you need to be convinced, right? **Studies show** that eating dark chocolate in moderation (like two servings a week) is associated with a lower risk of heart failure. Why? Dark chocolate is very high in antioxidants and provides essential minerals and some fiber as well. The fats contained in the dark chocolate are of the healthier sort – mostly monounsaturated fats.

Chocolate might also have a mildly positive effect on blood pressure due to the flavanols content. In some studies, it has been shown to help protect against the harmful effects of LDL cholesterol and to boost the effects of HDL cholesterol.

There is one catch though – not just any chocolate will do. You need to look for dark chocolate that has a cacao content of at least 70-80%. One serving is around about an inch square so you cannot eat the whole slab. The advantage of dark chocolate over the cheaper brands is that it is very rich – you will be satisfied with a smaller serving size.

It is also not quite as sweet so you will be less inclined to eat as much of it. This is a sinfully delicious diet food – you feel as though you are cheating but this is one "cheat" that actually has good health benefits.

ACTION PLAN

- Find a good quality dark chocolate – Belgian chocolate is a good place to start.

- If you battle with portion control when it comes to chocolate, only buy a small slab at a time. Break it into single portion pieces and freeze individually – only take out one piece at a time. This will make it easier to prevent you from overdoing it.

Everyday Habit #123

Try to Be Happier

Having a sunny disposition is not only likely to make you more popular, it is also likely to help you live longer. Those that are really happy have been found to cut their risk of dying prematurely by a third, **according to a 2012 study**.

Happiness is very good for you and it's not just because you are likely to be more optimistic. When you are happy it is easier to cope with stress and your body produces less cortisol. Your blood pressure is also less likely to be raised.

Both of these factors combine to lower your risk of having a heart attack or stroke. The good news is that you can, to a large extent, learn to be happy. Changing the way you look at things can go a long way to help you feel more satisfied and fulfilled.

Be Grateful for What You Have

You can choose to be envious of what other people have but that will not make you happier as a person. Learning to look at what you have got in your life, as opposed to what you lack, and being grateful for that is just one way to help you feel more satisfied with life in general.

It may seem like a cliché but there is always someone out there that is worse off than you are and it pays to remind yourself of that once in a while. We can get so caught up in the struggle to acquire new things and what we will have in the future that we forget to enjoy what we do have in the present.

Find Out What You Really Want

Many of us go through life doing things that are expected of us rather than things that we things that we want to do. Sometimes the problem is that we don't even know what it is that we want ourselves.

Start out by giving this some serious thought. What is it that you are passionate about? If time and money were not an issue, what is it that you would do? These are just a few of the questions that you should be asking yourself to figure out what you really want from life. It could take you some time to find out what you really do want. Sometimes we set goals only to achieve them and find out that they are not what we expected or that our priorities have changed.

Finding your bliss can be a lifelong process but it is a very worthwhile one. If you can find out what you were put on this earth to do and can figure out a way to make a living at that, you will be truly happy. Working will no longer seem like a chore but will be something that you look forward to every day. Isn't that worth spending some time on?

Incorporate What You Love

Now that you have a better understanding of what it is that you are passionate about, find ways to start including that in your life. Maybe your dream is to have a book published – why not set aside time every day or second day to write? Find something that makes you happy – something that you want to do and find ways to incorporate it into your life, every day, if possible. That is the way to a more satisfying life. Maybe you feel as though you are in a dead-end job at the moment – incorporating something that you are passionate about into your life will help you to get some happiness despite the job and, who knows, you may even come up with a way to make money doing what you love.

Be Kind to Someone Every Day

Doing good things helps to uplift us. Look for opportunities to be kind to others every day – to strangers as well as those that you love – it is a great way to feel better about yourself. Smile at someone in the street, help someone carry their groceries. Volunteer at a local charity. The more you help others, the better you will feel about yourself and the happier you will be in your own life. It is not hard to find nice things to do for people, even strangers.

ACTION PLAN

- Start by getting yourself a little diary and keep it by your bed. Every morning and evening, write down 5-10 things that you are grateful for – these could be something as simple as a letter that came in the mail or as big as landing your dream job. The point of this exercise is to show you that you have a lot to be grateful for. The old adage, "Count your blessings" is very sage advice.

- Figure out what it is that you would ideally like to earn money doing. If you are not sure, think back to things that you enjoyed doing as a child. Is there any way to make these dreams a reality?

- Identify small steps that you can take today towards living your dream.

Everyday Habit #124

Get on Your Feet

Many of us have jobs that mean that we sit in front of a computer all day – these can swell your bank account but they can also swell your body. **Research shows** that women who sit for over six hours a day are about 40% more likely to die prematurely for any reason than women who spend less than 3 hours a day seated, irrespective of fitness levels.

Talk to your boss about getting that standing desk or look for ways to get on your feet more often throughout the day. Make a point of standing at least once every twenty minutes or so – perhaps you can stand while making calls. Carry this behavior over into your home life as well. Make a point of getting off the couch and doing something that is more active. Anything that gets you off the couch and moving is really going to be good for you.

If you take the average woman today and look at her counterpart 100-200 years ago, you will find that the general fitness levels have declined. This sedentary lifestyle that we have imposed on ourselves is a fairly new invention. 100 years ago, your average women would take a fairly brisk daily walk, possibly ride a horse, worked in the kitchen and garden and socialized a good deal more. For all the wonders of the technological age, we are actually a lot more stressed out than ever before, and our health is suffering for it.

ACTION PLAN

- Find ways to incorporate more activity into your day – go over to your colleague's desk to deliver a message rather than phoning it through or emailing it to them. Increased activity is good for your productivity overall.

- Is there some way that you can find to spend at least an hour a day on your feet? Instead of spending your lunch hour behind your desk, why not take a walk instead?

Everyday Habit #125

Don't Overeat

According to Dan Buettner, an author who has studied longevity across the globe, the oldest Japanese people tend to stop eating when they are around about 80% full. They never eat everything on their plates. If you want to live to be 100, leaving a little bit of food on your plate may be a good idea. Studies conducted in 2008 by researchers in St Louis have established that you can slow the aging process by eating less.

By consuming fewer calories, you are decreasing the amount of T3, a thyroid hormone, that your body produces. T3 is one of the hormones responsible for making you age faster. More and more studies are finding that regular fasting can also be beneficial. There is a school of thought that we should only eat two meals a day, rather than the three that most of us base our diets around.

The thinking is that in evolutionary terms, we were never meant to have so much food at our disposal all the time. Early man had to rely on his skills as a hunter and gatherer and so there would have been times of scarcity and times of plenty. Contemporary western society seems to be stuck in times of plenty. If fasting seems like too much for you to handle, you can still benefit by cutting down on the number of calories that you consume. If you have started following some of the other tips in this book, like increasing your intake of fruit and vegetables and cutting back on red meat consumption, you should already be eating less calories every day.

ACTION PLAN

- Aim to leave around about 20% of the food on your plate. We have been raised to view this as wasteful but think about the potential benefits in terms of longevity in order to motivate yourself. Just do not increase the size of the portions to compensate!

- Look at what you eat on a daily basis. Is that afternoon snack really necessary? Do you need to eat such a big meal for supper?

- Are there any empty calories that you can cut out? Even cutting out one cup of coffee or a can of soda a day can help – there must be something that you can cut back on.

I hope you have learned something from this book so far and would greatly appreciate it if you could leave an honest review on Amazon.com.

Everyday Habit #126

Have "Fun" Time – Regularly!

Having satisfying sex two to three times per week can add as many as three years to your life. Getting busy can burn an impressive amount of calories—sometimes as much as running for 30 minutes – and it is a lot more fun as well. (Which would you rather do?)

Regular sex may also lower your blood pressure, improve your sleep, boost your immunity, and protect your heart. It is a great way to work on stress and to promote relaxation. It is a great way to get extra exercise without it feeling like work and is also a great way to improve intimacy levels with your spouse/ significant other.

Schedule "fitness" sessions for the two of you on a regular basis and you will find that you are both fitter and healthier for it. Scheduling sex may not seem like a very spontaneous thing to do but it may be necessary if the two of you are very busy. Look for fun ways to incorporate more sex into your lives. It may require that you rely on your support network more – get the kids out of the house and get busy.

ACTION PLAN

- How often do you and your partner have sex, really?

- Speak to them about ways to increase the frequency more – perhaps there are things that both of you would like to try to increase the excitement factor.

- Make sure that the logistics work – can you leave the kids with your mother once a week? Scheduling time for each other without the kids may be a great way to make this work.

Discover Scientifically-Proven "Shortcuts" & "Hacks" to Lose Weight FASTER (With Very Little Effort)

For this month only, you can get Linda's best-selling & most popular book absolutely free – *Weight Loss Secrets You NEED to Know*.

Get Your FREE Copy Here:
TopFitnessAdvice.com/Bonus

Discover scientifically-proven tips to help you lose weight faster and easier than ever before. With this book, readers were able to improve their weight loss results and fitness levels. So, it's highly recommended that you get this book, especially while it's free!

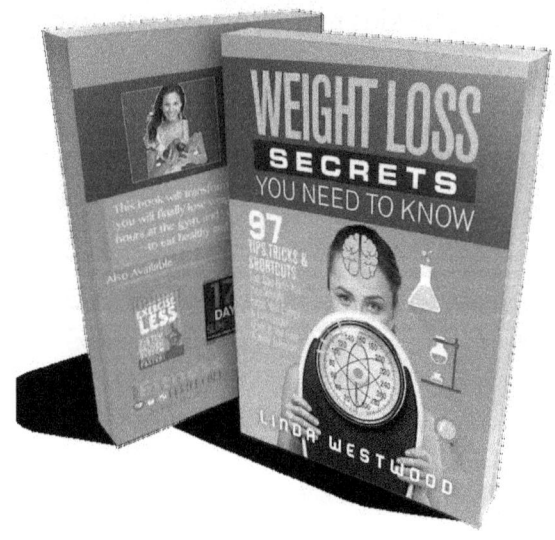

Get Your FREE Copy Here:
TopFitnessAdvice.com/Bonus

Conclusion

You have now read through all 126 healthy habits that can help you stick to a healthy diet and lose weight faster. Remember to take it a step at a time and track your progress. Achieving goals is just as much about appreciating how far you've come as it is about focusing on how far you have left to go.

It is also important to be prepared to make mistakes. The biggest and most worthwhile changes you make in your life don't come easily and they don't happen all at once. If you could perfectly adopt a new, healthy habit without making a single mistake or slip up, which would mean it was already a habit of yours to begin with.

So be prepared for slip-ups and don't let them bring you down and stop your progress. There will be days where it feels frustrating and difficult. You will want to give up. But these are exactly the days that will make you stronger. For each tough day you push through and each slip you get back up from, you will be that much stronger and that much closer to achieving your weight loss goals.

The stronger you get, the easier it will be to get through the next tough day. Your mistakes are not a sign of weakness. They are a sign that you are challenging yourself to do better. It's like exercise. If you've really pushed yourself during a workout, you're going to have sore muscles because the exercise has actually torn them. It's the process of repairing those tears that makes you grow stronger.

So, remember: it's the process of making mistakes and pushing past them that will give you the strength and will power you need to achieve your goals. Start practicing your new, healthy habits today and take pride in each step you take along the way!

Final Words

I would like to thank you for purchasing my book and I hope I have been able to help you and educate you on something new.

If you have enjoyed this book and would like to share your positive thoughts, could you please take 30 seconds of your time to go back and give me a review on my Amazon book page.

I greatly appreciate seeing these reviews because it helps me share my hard work.

You can leave me a review on Amazon.com.

Again, thank you and I wish you all the best!

Enjoying this book?

Check out my other best sellers!

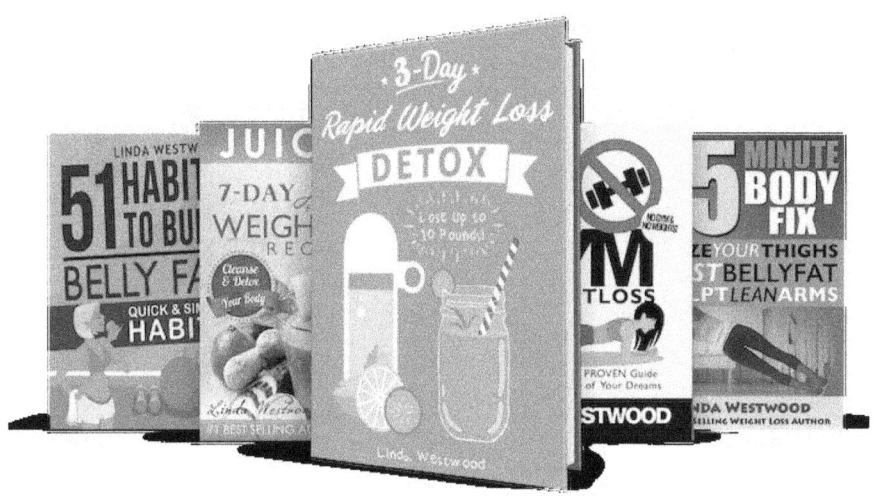

Get your next book on sale here:

TopFitnessAdvice.com/go/books

www.ingramcontent.com/pod-product-compliance
Lightning Source LLC
Chambersburg PA
CBHW031144020426
42333CB00013B/497